LOVE
YOUR
HAIR

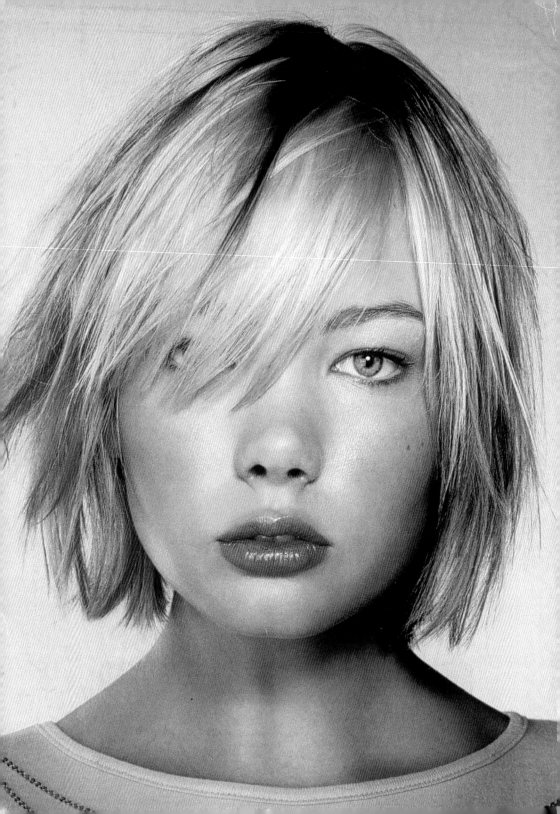

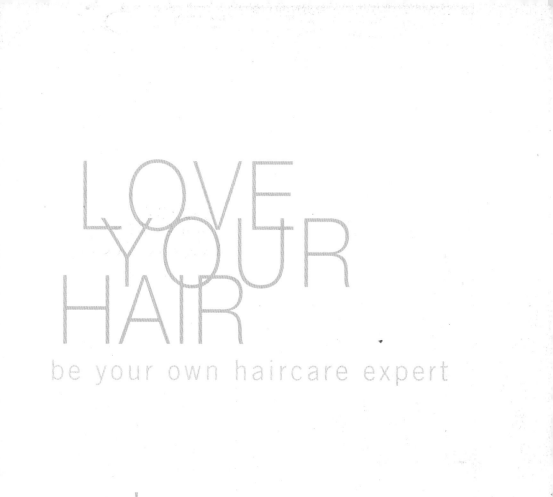

LOVE YOUR HAIR

be your own haircare expert

.andrew
jose

Thorsons

Thorsons
An Imprint of HarperCollins*Publishers*
77–85 Fulham Palace Road,
Hammersmith, London W6 8JB

The Thorsons website address is:
www.thorsons.com

and *Thorsons*
are trademarks of HarperCollins*Publishers* Ltd

First published by Thorsons 2002

10 9 8 7 6 5 4 3 2 1

© Andrew Jose 2002

Photography by Iain Phillpot, Tim Brett Day
Pantene photographs by kind permission of Proctor & Gamble
Studio photography by Robin Matthews
Illustrations by Margaret Hope
Hair and colour by Andrew Jose

Andrew Jose asserts the moral right to be
identified as the author of this work

A catalogue record of this book is
available from the British Library

ISBN 0 00 711900 3

Printed and bound in Italy by
Editoriale Johnson

308332

contents

thanks

My thanks go to my colleague David Cohen for helping me develop the concept of this book and for his good advice and support.

Special thanks to Su Clarke for her assistance and, to Ruth Cohen, without whose help I wouldn't have met my deadlines.

Thanks to the Andrew Jose team and the make-up artists and clothes stylists who have helped with the photography in this book.

Thanks to Proctor & Gamble for access to their Research and Development, and for their encouragement.

Thanks to Schwarzkopf International for their technical support on colouring and perming.

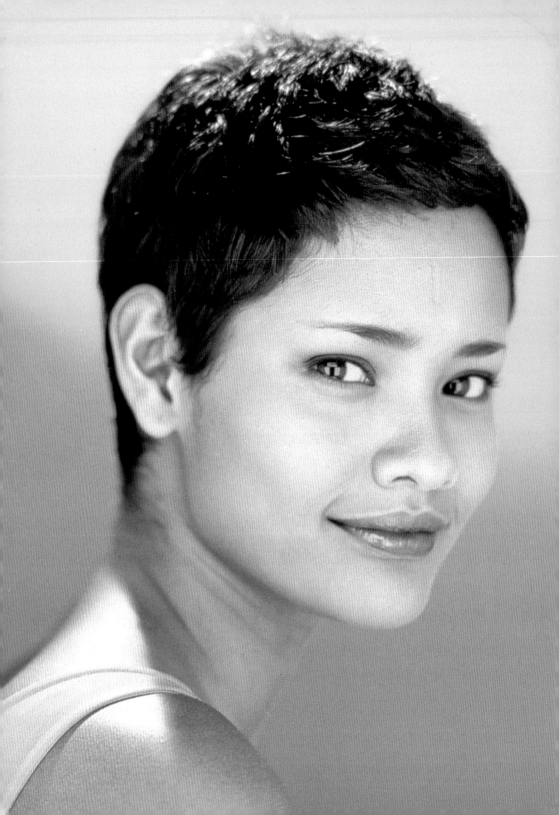

introduction

Enjoy your own haircare

It's been estimated that women spend an average of 45 minutes every day looking after their hair: washing, conditioning, perhaps colouring, certainly styling, putting it up, putting it down and tidying it on an evening out. And how about those 'bad hair days'? Why? Because it's important.

Every person's hair has great potential, but there are also limitations. This book will help you to achieve great results within these boundaries. It is my desire to answer as many of the questions that worry you and suggest solutions to your hair problems – based on the knowledge I have acquired caring for my clients over many years.

I would like you to enjoy caring for your own hair as much as I enjoy caring for my clients' hair. I would like you to be:

- happier with the results you achieve
- empowered with knowledge of your own hair
- sure of the products that will benefit your hair
- confident to style your hair.

Hair has always been important throughout history, even as far back as ancient times – just visit your local gallery and see the rich and famous from yesteryear. The Romans invented curling tongs; Cleopatra used henna to colour and condition her hair. In Japan, long before it opened its doors to the West, the women lacquered their hair – those Madam Butterfly looks didn't support themselves! Throughout the ages people have tried to change, alter, colour, curl or hide their hair under outlandish wigs. The opportunity to look and feel good has never been better than today.

Today the range of products and styling tools that are accessible and affordable would make our ancestors green with envy. Why, therefore, are so many people unhappy with their hair? They choose the wrong haircare regime, they worry about old wives' tales, feel they haven't got the skills to look after their hair and feel that it needs an inordinate amount of time to get good results.

I want to demystify the process for you and help you understand your hair, its needs, limitations and potential. This will enable you to choose the right products for your hair. I want you to be happier with the results and enjoy being your own haircare expert and not apologetic about looking after your hair.

love your hair

The key is knowing as much as you can about your own hair first – this is where this book starts. So let me help to empower you with knowledge. Take some time out for your hair – enjoy it and get the best results. *Love your hair.*

Andrew Jose

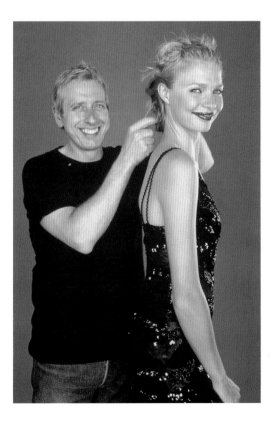

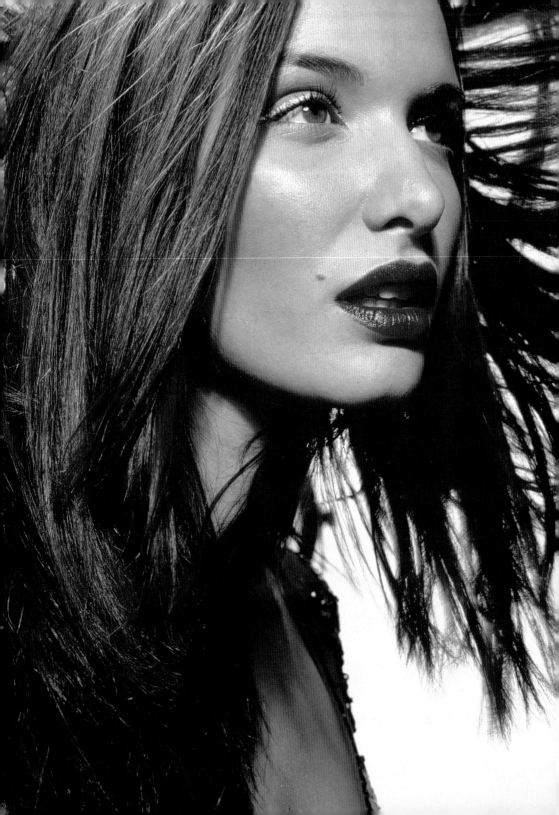

Hair isn't alive. In fact, as soon as hair breaks through the scalp it is dead.

know your hair

How many mornings have you looked in the mirror and thought, 'What am I going to do with my hair?' You know that any amount of primping isn't going to rescue it and make you feel good for the rest of the day. It sits limply on your head or flies in every direction. It won't respond to brushing, combing or styling. 'Why can't I control my hair? If only my bathroom cabinet came with a permanent hairdresser.'

The secret is to know your hair:

its type, its condition, what it can and can't do and the products and tools that will help. To banish morning hair blues, you really need to get in touch with your hair – then you'll love it.

Knowing your hair

The first thing I do when I give a consultation to a client, after seating them in front of a mirror, is to put my hands through their hair in order to feel, examine and get to know it. So take a little time out and really get in touch with your own hair. Run your fingers through it, feeling the hair and scalp, and examine individual hairs. Remember, your hands are an important partner in caring for your hair, so let the two get to know each other.

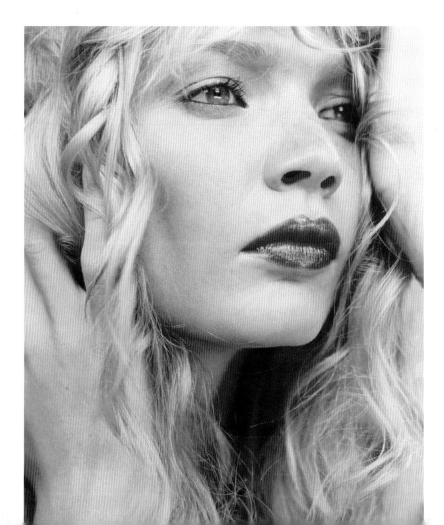

Hair isn't alive. In fact, as soon as a hair breaks through the scalp it is dead. The bulb at the bottom of the hair follicle is alive and causes the hair to continue to grow at a rate of around 1 cm (½ inch) every month. Hair is made up of keratin, the same protein that appears in our nails, skin and teeth. Unlike skin, hair cannot repair itself when it is damaged, so it is important to learn how to take care of your hair.

3 basic steps towards knowing your hair

There are three basic tests you can do whilst examining your hair that will teach you about its general state. They address the root, the hair and the condition. You should do this on clean, dry hair.

1. Carefully pull out a hair by placing a small tight-toothed comb close to the scalp and lifting it up as you run it through your hair. Check to see if the hair has a bulbous end. If it has, the hair is healthy. If it hasn't, your hair is unhealthy and is breaking.

2. Take a few strands of hair and run your thumb and forefinger along them. Start from the end near to the root. It may take a bit of practice, but eventually you will be able to feel where the texture of the hair changes. Often the condition changes as you move along the shaft, with the healthier hair nearer the root. You'll feel a sudden ridge and the hair will be drier towards the end. This is where you should apply conditioner.

3. Create a parting down the centre of your head and then with a fingertip lightly rub the skin in the parted area. Take a look at your fingertip. A sheen suggests oily hair, nothing suggests normal hair and flakes of skin suggest a dry scalp.

It is very important and useful to understand the basics of how your hair grows and is made up, especially when it comes to product use. Overleaf is a free drawing of an enlarged hair follicle and shaft.

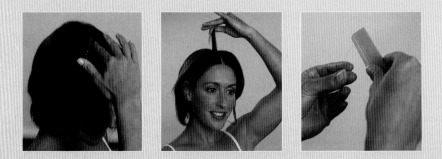

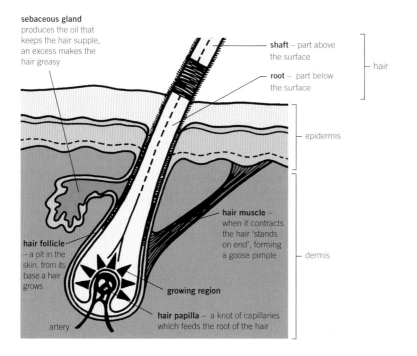

sebaceous gland produces the oil that keeps the hair supple, an excess makes the hair greasy

shaft – part above the surface

root – part below the surface

hair

epidermis

hair muscle – when it contracts the hair 'stands on end', forming a goose pimple

dermis

hair follicle – a pit in the skin, from its base a hair grows

growing region

artery

hair papilla – a knot of capillaries which feeds the root of the hair

The cuticle

The cuticle is the outer covering of the hair shaft. It is like the bark of a tree and is important in protecting the cortex (the protein fibres that make up the bulk of the hair). In healthy hair the cuticles lay flat and over-lay each other. This gives the shine, as light is reflected on the smooth surface.

However, if the cuticle is raised, the hair becomes dull. It will also become tangled with other hair shafts. The cuticle then becomes worn and falls away, leaving the cortex exposed, which results in splits, breakage and exposure to pollution. Remember that this cannot be repaired. You just have to wait for new hair to grow. Correct conditioning can help to avoid further deterioration and tangling.

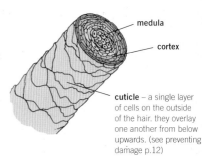

medula

cortex

cuticle – a single layer of cells on the outside of the hair. they overlay one another from below upwards. (see preventing damage p.12)

We lose about 100 hairs every day, but don't worry, the average head has between 100,000 and 140,000 hairs.

stages of growth

Baby

A baby's hair is soft and downy when it's born, and will often fall out.

Toddler

Toddlers have soft delicate hair, known as vellus, which has the same texture as the hair on our arms and body.

Child

Children's hair becomes coarser as they get older.

Teenager

The hair becomes much coarser on the scalp as well as eyebrows and lashes. It's also the time when underarm and pubic hair appears.

Adult

Our hair is fixed by the time we reach early adulthood and will remain that way unless there are changes to health and lifestyle.

Middle age

Grey hair can start appearing as the hair shaft loses pigment. Men may also experience baldness.

Elderly

Men may go bald, but women's hair should remain as thick as it was in adulthood unless ill-health or genetics is a factor.

Know your hair type

The first thing to be aware of is whether your hair is straight, curly, coarse, fine or a combination of these types. This is determined by your genetic make-up. European hair varies from straight to curly, while the colour ranges from dark brown to white blond. Afro hair is usually tightly curled and dark brown, whereas East Asian hair tends to be straight, thick, coarse and black. Aside from these general categories, there are even more variations in mixed races.

Hair twisters

All hair, even apparently straight hair, twists as it grows. The more twists there are in a given length of hair determines how curly it is. Afro hair has nearly twelve times as many twists as Caucasian hair.

The hair bulb mainly determines how curly the hair is. If the bulb lays to one side of the follicle, the hair will grow at an angle, or if there are variations in the bulb, the hair will twist more.

Texture

Much of the attraction of a beautiful head of hair lies in its texture, or feel. The texture of hair depends on several things.

1   The average diameter of the individual hairs. These vary widely. The larger the hair diameter, the coarser it will feel.
2   Different people's hair naturally feels different: some dry, some soft, some silky and others wiry. The reasons underlying these differences are still a matter for scientists to argue over.
3   The texture can be affected by weathering of the hair.

Oily hair

This is due to too much sebum being produced. Whatever the length of your hair, your scalp will produce the same amount of oil. This could be an inherited characteristic or caused by lifestyle and diet. Sebum must be washed away regularly because it can build up and make the hair lank and clump together.

Dry hair

As well as feeling dry, it is dull, sometimes frizzy, and gets tangled or breaks easily. It simply doesn't contain enough moisture, which could be due to a lack of sebum, the age of the hair, over-use of heat or chemical treatments or incorrect use of styling tools. The cuticles have opened up and the cortex has lost its moisture.

Normal hair

This is enviously soft yet strong, easy to handle, looks good most of the time and has lots of body. It has never been coloured or permed and the minimum amount of heat has been used. This sort of hair rarely needs to be conditioned.

Combination hair

This is probably one of the most common hair types. The scalp is greasy and the hair shaft is dry. It means that not only does it look lank and flat, but it also manages to be dull, lacklustre and flyaway looking.

Fine/flyaway/fragile hair

This is one of the most frustrating hair types as it can be quite difficult to control. Static is often caused by a dry atmosphere or the hair being in contact with synthetic fibre in a pillow or bedsheet. A second common characteristic is lack of volume. This type of hair needs careful grooming.

Tight curls

The hair is often fine and needs special care to look its best. It cannot be brushed and should only be combed when wet. When the curls are perfectly groomed without frizz the hair can be the most admired of all hair types.

Grey hair

This can affect people of all ages, but primarily as they get older. The loss of colour is due to the gradual fall in the melanin production in the hair bulb – grey hair is a mixture of hair with and without colour. Grey hair tends to be coarser. It may also absorb pollution which can cause the hair to appear yellow.

Hair concerns

Despite the uniqueness of everyone's hair, it is surprising how many people share the same concerns. Having cared for and styled the hair of thousands of clients from all parts of the world over the years, I am fascinated by the similarities of their worries. So I think it would be helpful to address these major concerns which are listed overleaf.

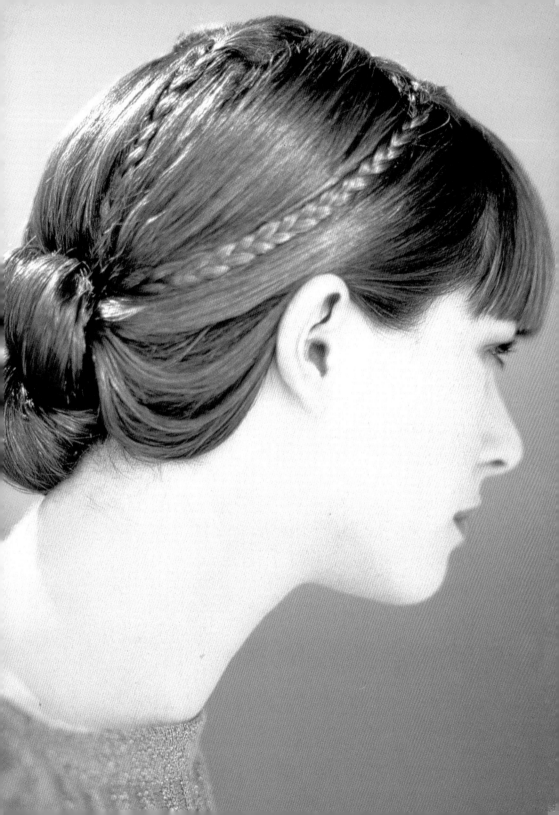

Damage

Damaged hair has three characteristics: the hair is dull or lifeless; it doesn't shine and it is difficult to manage.

Causes of damage

Weathering is apparent on older hair. Remember your hair grows at one centimetre a month so if you have shoulder-length hair, the ends will be at least two years old. Weathering is caused by wetting, friction, swimming, sunlight, colouring and perming. The most obvious sign is split ends.

Damage from the hairdresser

Blunt scissors, razors and sharp combs will affect the condition of your hair. Blunt scissors and razors give a jagged end to the hair which will make the cuticle susceptible to damage. Sharp combs used on wet hair may over-stretch the hair as it is at its most vulnerable when wet.

Permanent colour and perms

Any chemical procedure changes the hair. The hair has its structure disrupted or even changed in order to allow the colour to become permanent. Perming breaks the structure of the hair. The skills of the hairdresser who is neutralizing or restructuring the hair will be key to its quality after perming.

Condition, condition, condition. Prevention is better than cure.

Preventing damage

Keeping hair flexible with a high moisture content is the key. Use the finger test to determine the condition of your hair. Apply conditioner by massaging the dry area of the hair shaft so as to help push the conditioner into the hair, smoothing the cuticle along the hairshaft. Running your fingernail down the hair will also help smooth rough or raised cuticles. Always condition. Conditioner which is not needed will be rinsed away. Modern conditioners that are not oil-based will leave your hair full of life.

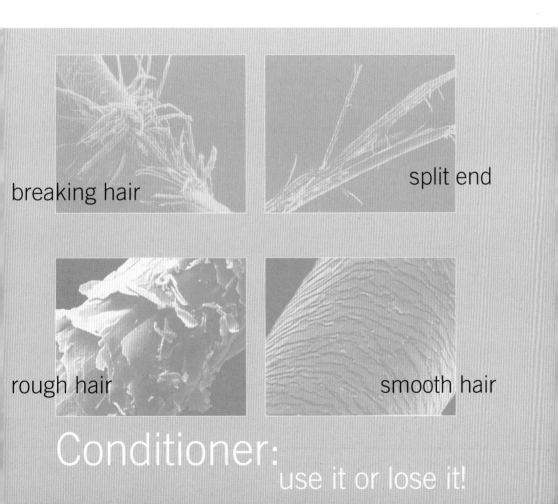

breaking hair

split end

rough hair

smooth hair

Conditioner: use it or lose it!

Sunfade

Many of us consider sunfade to be our greatest hair concern. Expensive colours can be ruined in a very short time with rapid fading.

Natural hair will be lightened quickly in strong sunlight and the hair will dry and fade. For many of us our two-week sunshine holiday will create the winter blues of poor hair condition.

Protecting hair in the sun

Covering the hair works, but it is not always practical. A good step is to use UV protection products, the Kerastase UV range is particularly effective in my experience.

Many products claim UV protection, yet unlike suntan lotion they give no indication of their effectiveness.

When sunbathing, apply conditioner to the hair regularly, particularly before swimming. Wet your hair in the shower and cover it with conditioner. Do not rinse it out, but reapply it when you reapply your suntan lotion.

Flyaway hair

Hugely frustrating, it usually affects finer hair types. It is caused by your environment: air conditioning, synthetic pillows and nylon hairbrushes. A build up of static electricity in your body will also create this problem.

Controlling flyaway hair

Conditioners that use Dimethicone, will help. This is a silicone compound made from silica, one of the commonest substances on earth.

These micro-fine droplets make the hair smooth and shiny, adding control to the hair by conditioning it. Blow-dry lotion is a very effective styling aid which will give general control. Smoothing a silk scarf over the hair will reduce static.

the essential kit for Holiday hair

- shampoo
- conditioner and treatment
- sun protector spray or inexpensive conditioner for beach use
- large toothed comb
- a travel hairdryer
- brush

Frizzy hair

This is a natural condition. There is a fantastic range of products available to help. The key is to decide how you wish your hair to be when finished, as this will influence your choice of shampoo and styling aids.

Smooth and straight

If perfect, straight hair is your chosen look, then the first step is to use frizz-reducing shampoo and conditioner. This is followed by a blow-dry lotion for straightening hair. Mousse is best for fine hair, whereas a serum or oily gel is best for frizzy hair types. Blow-dry with a bristle brush (Mason and Pearson) or a round type, and consider using straightening irons to give a catwalk finish.

Formed curls and waves

Shampoo and condition with frizz-reducing products. Comb through your hair and squeeze all excess water from the hair. Recomb it and then gently lift the hair from the bottom up, encouraging curls of waves to form. Apply a mousse or a light gel with the fingertips, moving from root to tip on each curl or wave. Very coarse hair will need a gel with an oil or silicon content. Apply. Allow the hair to dry naturally or gently use a dryer with a diffuser attachment. Avoid touching your hair as this will bring back the frizz.

it's natural for curly or wavy hair to frizz – and the look can be effective, but most of us are looking for ways to escape frizz

love your hair

Lack of body

Hair that lies flat and limp is an agony for many at some time or other. The cause is often to do with hair type, but it can also be due to inappropriate washing, bad cutting and a lack of general care. You need to carefully assess the products you use and how you treat your hair.

Body building

Avoid 2-in-1 and moisturizing shampoos. Choose a clarifying shampoo or one that promises volume. Try a new approach to blow-drying – dry the hair upside down and brush volume into it. Use styling products such as root-boosting mousses and gels to hold the volume. Try Velcro rollers, remembering that the longer your hair, the larger the roller should be.

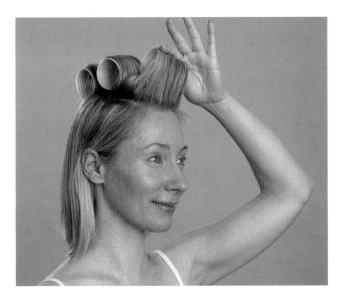

large velcro rollers are an easy way to create volume

Humidity

Humidity is one of the most frustrating spoilers of a good hair style. The warm moisture in the air dampens the hair and collapses the style, making it look limp and sad. However, there are aids to reduce this problem.

Light perms designed for blow-drying create hold and control, giving permanent lift to the hair. They will fare well in the most humid conditions. Using alcohol-based blow-dry lotions will create a dry hold. Finish all styles with a firm hairspray.

Healthy scalp

Having a healthy scalp, like all parts of the skin is important. Nothing is more unpleasant than having loose skin mix with the roots of the hair. Although dandruff is the most common scalp concern, there are scalp disorders such as psoriasis or infections like ringworm. I go into this in more detail later on in the book.

Scalp care

Regular washing and scalp massage will keep your scalp healthy. Dandruff is easily treated with readily available shampoos.

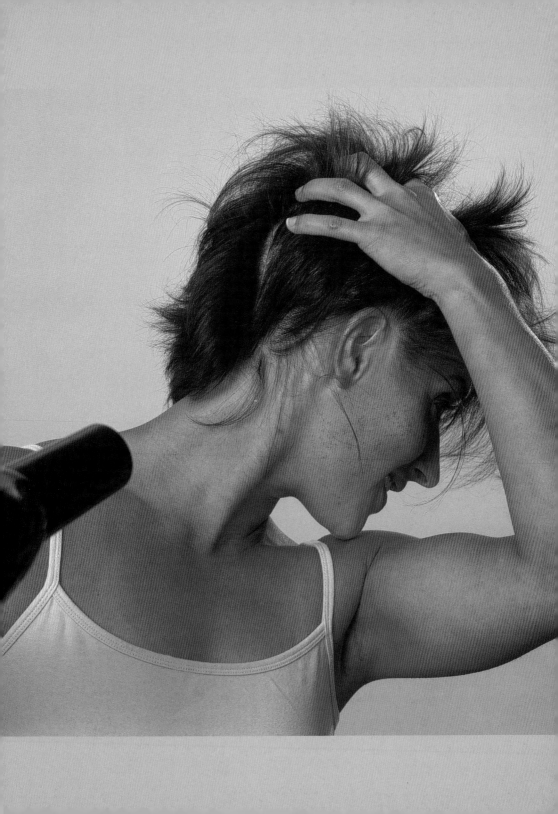

Hair concerns and solutions

Problem	Cause
hair loss	Multiple: diet, mineral deficiency, stress, genetic
dull	Product overload
brittle, dry	Over-processed, chlorine, sun
flat hair	Product overload, bad haircut
dandruff	Overproduction of yeast
split ends	Damaged hair through chemicals, brushing wet
flyaway	Static, lack of condition
infestation	Lice jumping from head to head
frizzy	Over-processing, humidity

Solution	Keywords to look out for on product
Visit your doctor or trichologist. They may recommend hormone treatments, better nutrition or mineral supplements	Hair loss
Revise wash plan and don't leave conditioner on for too long	Shine
Condition and specific treatment	Moisture, deep or intensive conditioning
Try new conditioning, leave on for shorter time	Volume
Dandruff treatment	Anti-dandruff
Regular hair cuts and try using a serum when dry	Strength
Avoid brushing it as much as possible, use a leave-in conditioner and use a styling product to give you control	Anti-static
Chemical lotions formulated for lice, or regular combing with nit comb	Pharmacist for solution
Always use styling products to tame the frizz, and condition hair regularly	Controls frizzy hair

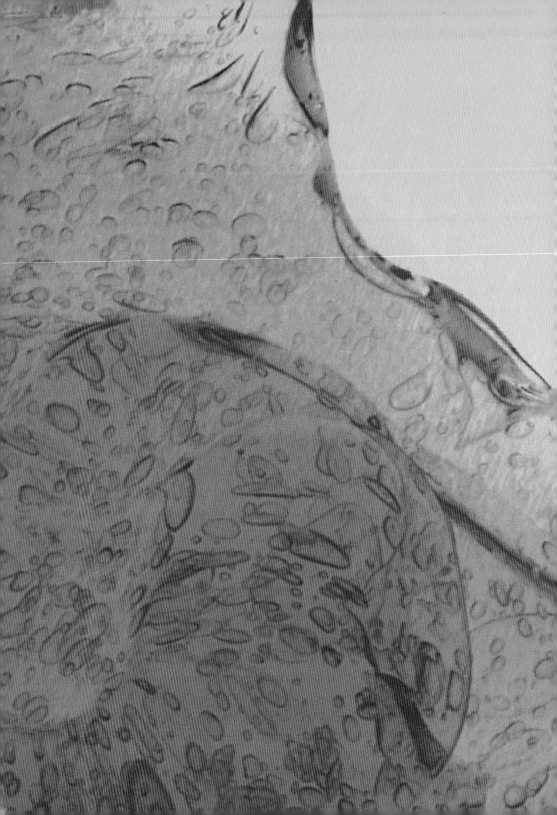

Nowadays, there is such a vast array of products to choose from. It can be confusing and even intimidating.

cleaning, conditioning, controlling

So should you use a shampoo for chemically-treated hair, or should you use a repair shampoo or perhaps a product developed especially for curly hair? Then there's the dilemma of how often you should wash your hair. Should you opt for a daily cleanser or a mild shampoo?

Shampoos contain surfactants which clean the hair by lifting off the excess sebum and dirt that has accumulated in the hair. They produce foam (lather), which holds the bits of dirt and stops them from being redeposited on the hair. The two most commonly used chemicals in shampoos are ammonium lauryl sulphate and ammonium laureth sulphate, which is milder. Mild shampoos are important for those with sensitive skin or for frequent washing. There are other ingredients in shampoos: fragrance to make it pleasant to use and volumizers and conditioning agents like Panthenol to make the hair feel smoother and thicker.

Choosing the ideal shampoo for your hair

This is often a case of trial and error. You have to work out what sort of hair you have and then consider other aspects, such as how often you wash your hair.

According to the experts you can't wash your hair too much. Most of the products that you use are washed away and won't sit on the scalp or hair if you rinse it thoroughly. Nor will washing too often trigger the sebaceous glands to suddenly start producing more sebum. However, it can wash away the sebum, which protects the hair, so if you like washing your hair most days then you will have to use a conditioner to replace the lost sebum. As for the type of shampoo to use, there are a variety of types to choose from.

Gentle shampoo

It may be worth trying a gentle shampoo that uses mild surfactants if you do wash frequently or have a sensitive scalp. A gentle formula may also work well for extra fine hair, or you could opt for a volumizing version that will puff up the hair shaft.

Moisturizing shampoo

If your hair is dry and brittle, coloured or permed, or simply very long and with ends that are more than a couple of years old, then you might find a moisturizing shampoo replenishes the hair and adds volume. Look out for shampoos aimed at chemically-treated hair.

Coloured hair

Colour fade is the biggest concern of all who colour their hair. As most colour fade happens by wetting the hair, almost nothing can be done to reduce this. Shampoos that are specially designed for coloured hair, moisturize the hair, stopping it from becoming dry after being chemically treated. Using a shampoo with a colour additive will delay the fading and keep the hair bright, as you are redepositing a little colour each time you shampoo. Shampoos for blond hair will neutralize any 'green' that may come from pollution. Your hair will be brighter and appear blonder. The product I use in my salon is KMS Blond Shampoo.

Permed hair

Perming, as with most chemical processes, dries the hair. Therefore a perm shampoo will give elasticity to the perm. If however, you cannot find a perm shampoo, use a good moisturizing shampoo at least once a week.

Greasy formula shampoo

Greasy hair will need a strong formula to lift the dirt and sebum that collects in the hair. It will work on the roots without drying out the longer hair. It will help give body to the hair and, by controlling the build up of sebum, prevent the dullness that greasy hair often has.

Deciding on the hair you *want* will make choosing your haircare product easier. For example, if your hair is fine and limp and you want volume, look for volume products rather than fine-hair products.

Anti-dandruff shampoo

Those of you who suffer from dandruff may need an anti-dandruff formula with anti-bacterial or anti-fungal agents. You can read more about dandruff in the chapter on hair solutions, so I won't go into great depth about it here. But don't worry about using a specialist shampoo, it won't damage your hair, it will merely work against the bacteria that causes your scalp to itch and help reduce the flaking caused by overproduction of yeast.

Clarifying shampoo

Another variety of shampoo that has crept onto the shelves in a big way recently is clarifying shampoo. Clarifying shampoo is more acid-based than the previous examples (although all shampoos are slightly acid to counter the alkaline of the hair) and is good for stripping your hair of the product build-up that can flatten and dull your hair. Using it once a month will help increase shine and volume.

If you are still a bit bemused about which shampoo to use why not talk to your hairdresser. Their advice is free.

Swimming shampoo

Finally there is the swimming shampoo aimed at you sporty types who frequently submerge yourselves in chlorinated swimming pools or salty sea water. Swimming plays havoc with the hair. The hair can get very dry and brittle, losing its shine and elasticity. Using a specialist shampoo every time you go swimming will help prevent the drying effect and bring back shine. Applying a conditioner to wet hair before swimming helps prevent chlorine entering the hair shaft.

Dry shampoos

Bahshe by Schwarzkopf is a readily available dry shampoo that is a session-hairdresser's secret. It's great to use when you don't have time for a shampoo or you are up a mountain doing a photo shoot. It is a powdery substance that absorbs natural oils or excessive products, leaving hair with a slightly dusty appearance. A fine talcum powder could also be used in emergencies or for dusty-looking catwalk styles.

Shampooing your hair

There is a right way and a wrong way to wash hair. When your hair is wet it is at its most vulnerable. Rough treatment can cause breakages and tangles, so be careful.

- **Always wash your hair under a flow of water,** preferably standing under a shower or hanging your head over the edge of the bath.

- **When you add the shampoo, work it into a lather** (it's the lather that helps lift off the dirt) by gently massaging your scalp.

- **Avoid digging your fingers into your scalp** and clawing away at your hair, it could get tangled.

- **Gently work the lather through the hair length.** Don't rub the hair, instead draw the shampoo through to the ends. This avoids disrupting the cuticles too much.

- **Finally, rinse the shampoo off thoroughly,** keeping the flow of water constant through the hair as it hangs down.

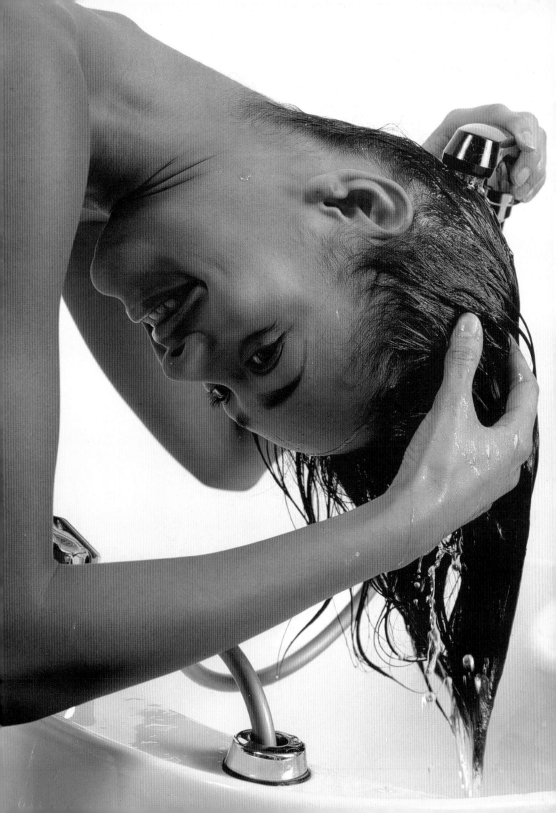

Never rub your hair with the towel. This can cause abrasive damage. Simply squeeze the excess water out and then wrap the towel around your head for five minutes or so to blot up the water.

Choosing your conditioner

A good conditioner complements your shampoo and is an essential support to your haircare regime. If you wash your hair daily, you need a light conditioner to replace the natural oils on the hair shaft.

The majority of conditioners don't repair hair damage (see note on cuticles). They prevent further damage and improve the appearance by smoothing the damaged cuticle, making it shinier and easier to maintain. Conditioners do this by coating the hair shaft and making the cuticle lie flat. They aren't absorbed into the hair shaft because they need to do their job on the outside. Once the cuticle is flattened the hair will be shinier and easier to comb. Conditioners also help combat flyaway hair by reducing the static electricity of the hair.

Conditioning falls into two categories: moisture and strength.

Generally, fragile hair needs strengthening and dry hair needs moisture. But some hair will need both.

Intensive treatment

For those with dry and brittle hair, and spilt ends, you should combine an intensive treatment into your grooming regime once a month. These add strength by depositing protein molecules into the cuticles.

Volumizing

Volumizing conditioners puff up the hair shaft by clinging on and making it appear fuller, which is great for fine hair.

Leave-in formulas

Other forms of conditioning include leave-in formulas, which are good for those who always blow-dry because they protect the hair from heat damage. They are also less time-consuming if you wash your hair every day.

taking extra time when conditioning can radically improve the quality of the hair.

If you find your hair gets greasy more quickly than usual, then your conditioner could be too heavy. But rather than throw it away and start again, try rinsing it off sooner and for a little longer. If it continues to get greasy, move onto another brand.

Conditioning your hair

When conditioning, unlike shampooing, you can be selective with application. Taking these extra moments can radically improve the quality of the hair.

- Avoid putting conditioner on the roots. The hair is new and won't need to be conditioned. It could just make the hair lie flat against your head, reduce volume, clog the pores and leave little flakes in your hair like dandruff.
- Work it through the hair length carefully.
- **Never** brush wet hair. Gently comb the conditioner through to the ends.
- Leave it on for a couple of minutes, or longer for intensive treatments, but be careful, the longer you leave it, the more chance it will become over-conditioned which causes the hair to be heavy and lank.
- Rinse thoroughly, running water through the hair as it hangs down. Avoid rubbing it in case it gets tangled or the cuticles are lifted up.
- Blot with the towel as I described in the shampoo section and then gently comb through.

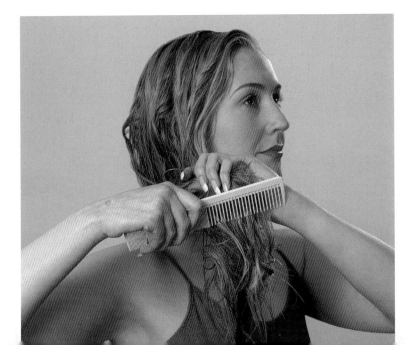

Scalp massages

In addition to being therapeutic, scalp massages are also good for the hair because they stimulate the blood flow to the hair follicles, encouraging the release of essential nutrients in the bulb. It's like a gym workout for the head. It will also loosen dead skin cells.

Simply spend a little more time when shampooing your hair and turn it into a special moment. Try doing it last thing at night before you go to sleep. You'll find it marvellously invigorating and it will help keep your hair healthy and strong. However you must be gentle to avoid damaging the hair, and if you have greasy hair, you may find massaging it too often stimulates the production of sebum.

The step-by-step massage I've designed for you to use at home can be used on wet or dry hair. It will relax and improve circulation and will also give some relief from tension headaches.

A tightness of the scalp can be relieved during your hair conditioning. You'll need 10 minutes for this exercise.

1 Run the conditioner through the hair until it feels slippery.

2 Place both hands on your head. Try to create a cap for the head by placing your thumbs behind the ears at the edge of the hairline. Spread your fingers to cover as much of the scalp as possible.

3 Exerting as much pressure as possible, move the fingertips in small circular movements.

4 Slowly move your hands around until all parts of the head have been massaged.

5 Using your fingertips and the same circular movements, move around the hairline from the forehead to the nape. When the fingers meet, move from the nape over the crown to the centre of the forehead. Massage the temples with your thumbs as you make this movement. Relax and enjoy.

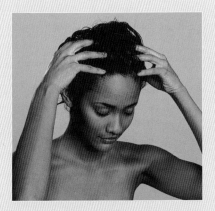 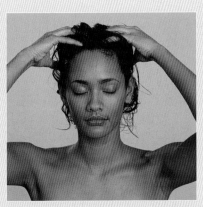

Styling aids

The most exciting recent advance in haircare that can help you avoid that bad hair day, is in the development of styling aids. You really have the potential now to control and style your hair everyday. Amazing names like Elastic, Sparkler and Twist inspire you, but the choice is becoming evermore challenging.

Gels, creams, mousses and sprays

There are different ways of applying styling aids – gels, mousses, wax, creams and sprays. You should have no preconceptions about the product performance or application, as these are purely methods of delivering the product.

It is the formulas in these products that will help you with your styling. The way you like your styling solution delivered will be your choice. It may be a combination. Opposite are my personal recommendations.

ensure the mousse is distributed evenly right down to the roots of your hair

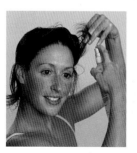 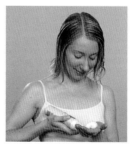 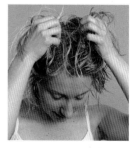

lift the hair up and spray root booster directly into your roots

Required result	Look for
Volume	Root-booster sprays, mousse for volume
Frizz control	Gels with oil content, serums
Clean curls	Sculpting lotions, curl-defining spray, Awapuhi mist
Hold	Hairsprays
Control in humid conditions	Blow-dry sprays, Hairspray
Smooth	Smoothing mousse
Strengthen	Strengthening serum – non greasy
Bed head	You'll know when you've found it – wax etc.
Choppy/definition	Definition creams, Kiehl's silk and groom

Essential tools

Hairbrushes

There are almost as many varieties of hairbrush as there are shampoos or conditioners, and each one has a valid reason to exist. Well, almost.

There's the paddle, the Denman classic, the Mason and Pearson and the vent brush. Then there are brushes for grooming, curling, volumizing and even some that use heat. Each one is devised for a particular hair type and finish.

Paddle brushes are great for detangling and smoothing long hair.

The **Denman classic** is used to add volume and polish during blow-drying.

Mason and **Pearson brushes** are also kind to the hair and good for brushing dry hair into smooth styles.

The purpose of the **curling brush** is to separate and define curls and to add in waves during blow-drying. The smaller the brush, the smaller the curl.

Vent brushes are designed to speed up blow-drying without damaging the hair by encouraging air to circulate underneath and around the brush while drying. And size does matter, the longer the hair the larger the brush should be.

Combs

Combs come in different shapes and sizes as well.

You will need a **large toothed comb** for when hair is wet or really curly, or for combing conditioner through the hair.

There's also the **tail comb** which is good for creating partings, dressing and separating hair.

You can also use **clips** to separate the hair off during drying, and **Velcro rollers** to add volume and shape to your hair.

Electrical tools

If used carefully, electrical grooming tools are brilliant for getting hair to do what you want. Straight hair can be texturized with crimpers or given waves with a **diffuser** attached to a hairdryer. Curls of all shapes can be conjured up by **curling tongs**, or flattened completely with a nozzled hairdryer and **straightening irons**.

Diffusers gently dry hair encouraging natural movement. Especially good for curly hair and keeps frizz to a minimum when using a hairdryer.

Heated tongs or irons can easily create waves and curls. The size of the section of hair you're working on will determine the size and shape of wave. (N.B. it does take time and they get very hot, so be careful.)

Straightening irons should be used with a protective spray suited to your hair type. Small sections will help your hair stay in shape longer.

However, you do have to be a bit careful as heat can easily damage hair. If you blow-dry your hair, tong or iron it regularly, use a mousse, gel or leave-in conditioner that will protect your hair from the heat.

Every Christmas a host of electrical and gas-fired appliances come onto the market. Some will be good and some will disappear forever after the January sales. The products I have listed are proven and are constantly being improved. Personal recommendation is your best guide.

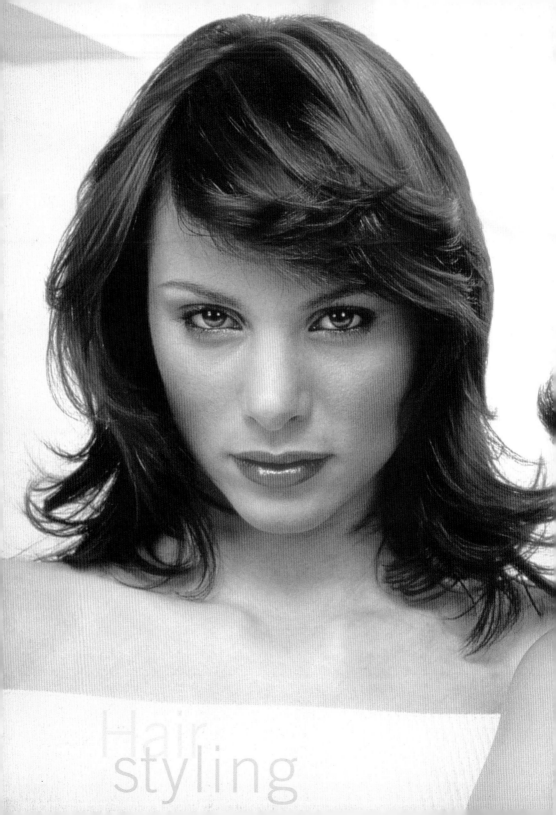

Hair
styling

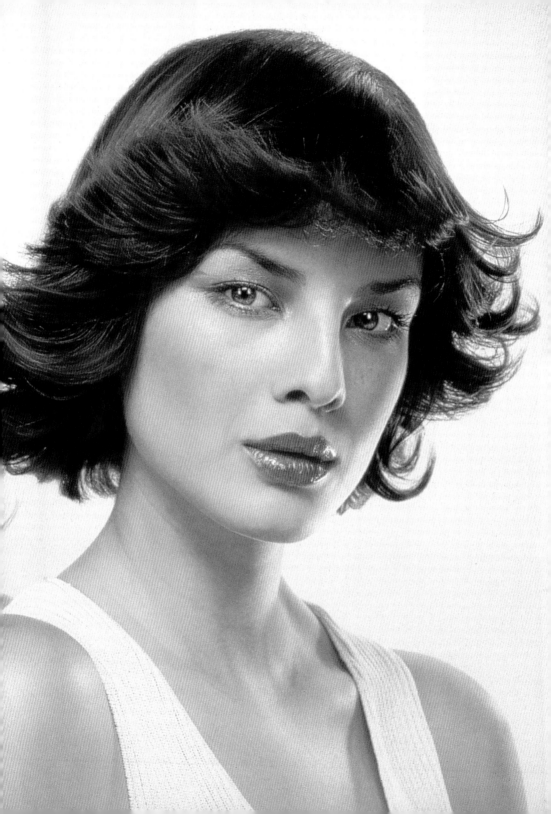

Blow-drying

The most important heated tool you can own is a hairdryer, so invest in a professional-style dryer with a long cylinder and an easy-to-hold handle. See how light it is compared to other models because you don't want to tire yourself out holding up a heavy one. Consider a diffuser and a nozzle, so you can create any style you want.

If you like sleek and shiny hair, use the nozzle attachment. It concentrates the air on a narrow section of your hair, pushing the cuticles flat. Never hold the dryer so that it blows up your hair shaft because this will lift every cuticle making your hair dull and prone to tangling.

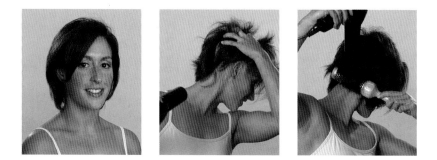

use your fingers to produce lift and movement into the roots

To add volume, tip your head upside down and blow the roots up. This is also the way to spike short hair.

To add texture, use the diffuser attachment and heap sections of the hair into the diffuser. The hot air will then dry it in a haphazard way, giving it lots of movement. If you have time, clip the hair up in sections so they cool and set in shape.

the added volume creates shape

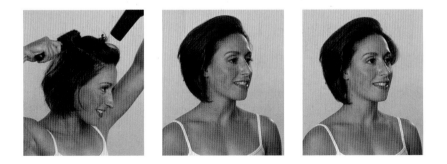

section the head and build volume into each area

Curling tongs

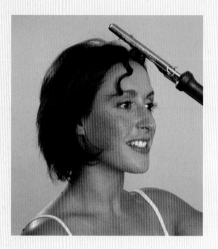

These come in all different sizes, and will give you curls galore. Some blow-dry hair like a hair-dryer, while others are solid metal cylinders that heat up. The gas-fired tongs are good for travelling. Always use a styling product that will hold the curl once it is formed, and don't drag the hair off the tongs. Slide it along so the curl stays intact, then fix it with a Kirby clip. Hair sets as it cools, rather than when it is hot, so always give it time to cool in position then your style will last longer.

from perfect curls
to smooth and sleek

Straightening irons

Treat these with care because you are literally ironing your hair. Always put a protector, like leave-in conditioner, on the hair and then slowly draw the irons down from the root to the end, keeping the irons moving and following the direction of the cuticle. It will make them lie flat and give the hair lots of shine.

Curling your hair with tongs takes practice, but it's worth persisting. They get very hot, so be careful!

Crimpers

You either love crimpers or hate them. The finish is so recognizably crimped, but it can be fun. You can get lots of different settings nowadays, allowing you to change the depth of the crimp. Some makes come with different attachments and can crimp and iron. Try putting your hair up in spiky bunches and crimping the ends for a funky effect.

Heated rollers

They are now back in fashion and perfect for volume, lift and movement. Buy the rollers without spikes on the barrel as they give a better finish to the hair.

Hot brushes

These are great for short- and medium-length hairstyles that need a lift throughout the day. Carry them in your bag and refresh your hair when needed.

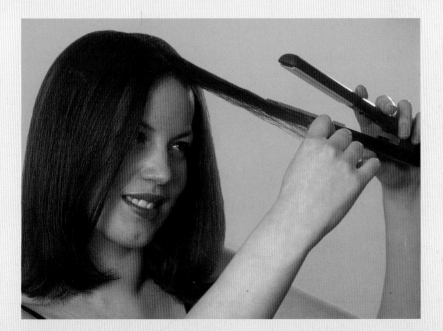

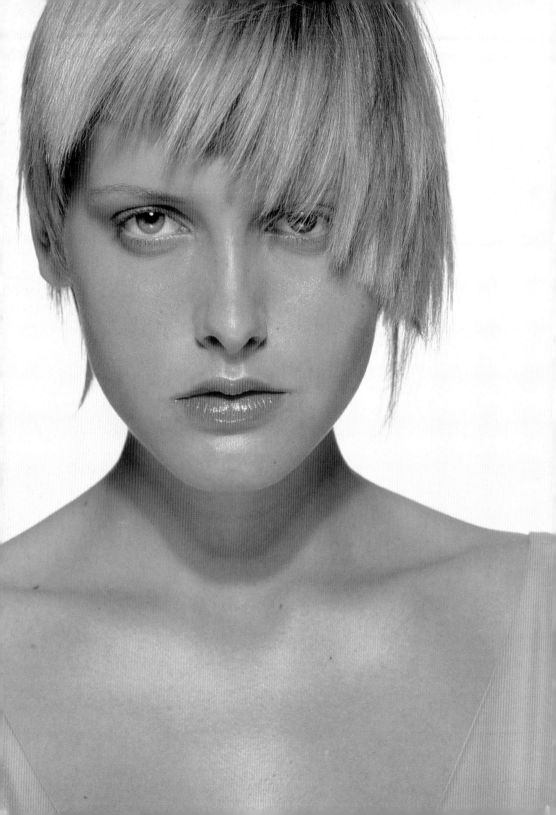

A good haircut is the foundation of your style and healthy hair.

your
haircut

A good haircut is the foundation of your style and healthy hair. It is also important to have the advice and benefit of an expert. Your hairdresser should be able to keep you abreast of the latest hair fashions and new products. They will have the eye to advise you on the style that will suit you and your lifestyle.

Your hairs grow at different rates so you will need to have a trim or restyle every six to eight weeks depending on the length, with short styles needing more upkeep than longer ones.

Finding a hairdresser

The first step is to go on recommendation. Ask your friends, especially if you like their hair. Or if you see someone in the street with nice hair, stop and ask them where they go. They will probably be flattered.

When looking for a new salon, consider booking a wash and blow-dry before taking the plunge with a haircut. This way you can have a risk-free taster of their service, and check out other people's cuts while you're there.

The next step is to build up a rapport with your stylist. Book up a consultation first (which should be free), so you can meet your stylist. This will give you both an opportunity to find out about one another and to see if you can trust him or her. It gives the stylist a chance to understand your lifestyle, the sort of hair you have and the expectations you hold. The first thing they'll need to establish is how much time you're prepared to give to the upkeep of your style. Honesty is crucial at this point for finding and keeping a good hairstyle. I always compare it to a New Year's resolution. Just remember how many times you make that promise, only to break it. Don't pledge yourself in the enthusiasm of the moment to keep to a routine which is not practical for you.

When you do finally go for your haircut, turn up on time and with reasonably clean hair. And at the end of the appointment tell the hairdresser what you honestly think. If you hate it, he or she will try to rectify it, and if you love it, he or she will appreciate being told.

- If you've found your perfect hairdresser, you don't want to lose them so make sure you always:

- Turn up on time.

- Never miss appointments without calling.

- Go with reasonably clean hair.

- Take a picture of what you would like.

- It is customary to tip 10–15% if you're happy with the service. Stipulating how the tip should be divided between the people who've served you is quite usual.

- Be willing to review your style occasionally.

- Try a bit of colour – you will look better with it.

- Don't rush your stylist – give yourself enough time to discuss the service you require and possibly have a change.

- If you like your hair, say so.

- If you don't, explain why.

- If you're concerned about not being attended to or your bleach having been left on too long, speak up – it does happen.

- If your stylist is finishing/drying your hair and you think you won't be able to do the same yourself, ask them to teach you.

- If your stylist recommends a new styling product, try it.

Listen to your hairdresser's opinion, but if you don't think something's right, then say so.

What's in a good haircut?

A good haircut doesn't just look good when you leave the salon. The things to consider are how it moves when you walk, how easy it is to maintain and keep it looking right and finally, how well it grows out. Your hairdresser should make it as easy as possible to maintain. Don't be afraid to ask for a blow-dry lesson.

But even if you do trust your hairdresser, would you still sit back and take no part in deciding what happens to your hair? No, I thought not. And it's important not to. You have to let your stylist know what you want. Taking pictures along with you when you are considering a radical change will help communicate your wishes and ideas, but knowing the language of hair-dressing helps even more.

There a few classic haircuts around and the different styles you see are usually variations on these. It makes it much easier for your hairdresser if you know the name of the sort of style you want.

If your hair needs lots of styling then apply mousse or gel spray before you rough dry and then add a smaller amount once it is 80% dry to achieve the final shape and definition you are looking for.

Modern classics

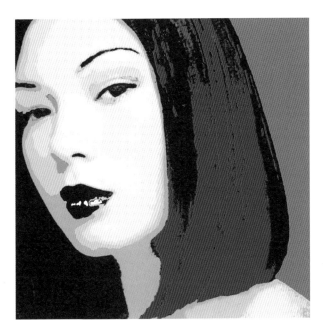

The bob

Straight, cut with scissors and precisely balanced, it is one of the most enduring styles around. It is high maintenance, requiring a daily blow-dry and monthly cut.

Style leaders: Anne Wintour, Editor, *American Vogue* and Mary Quant

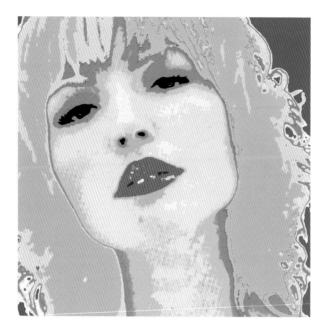

Shag/coup sauvage/shake

A layered haircut that is full of texture, ranging from 10 cm (4 inches) long to shoulder length. The tousled look needs only finger drying and funky styling products for definition. It is low maintenance, looks good as it grows out and needs cutting every 8 weeks.

Style leader: Courtenay Love

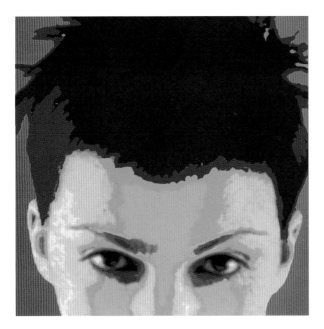

Pixie

This looks great with smaller faces and as women get older. It's a great way for the over '50s to look young. It is low maintenance, but needs cutting every 5 weeks.

Style leaders: Anne Robinson and Kate Moss

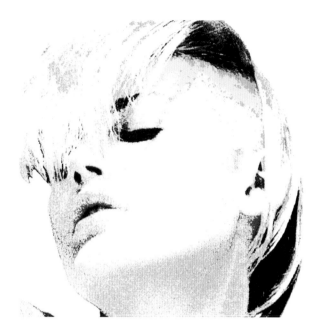

Buzz/undercut

Something for the young or forever young. The hair is cut short from the temples to the occipital bone (middle, back of head). The long hair on top covers the short hair and can be any length or style. The fun is that you can look different every day with the use of bobby pins, hair elastics and styling products. It needs to be cut every month to keep it closely cropped, but it looks great when it's growing out.

Style leaders: New York, London and Paris catwalk models

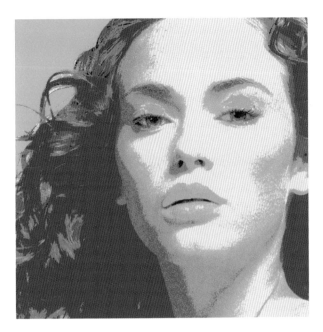

Pre-Raphaelite

This tends to be natural, as this sort of perming is not currently in vogue. Wavy hair is more sought after and achieved through encouraging natural kinks into waves with the use of styling products, tongs or diffusers. With straight hair the new perms can give this effect. Reasonably high maintenance.

Style leader: Jodie Kidd, international celebrity model (on the front cover of this book)

Hollywood hair

This is any hairstyle that requires a hairdresser's attention on a regular basis. Don't believe they just wash 'n' go!

Choosing your styles and varying your look is your choice, but you can't just take along a picture. The type of hair you have, its texture and the way it falls may be totally different from the hair you desire. It is rather like a scene from the film *Educating Rita* with Julie Walters. While she is still a hairdresser, Rita is asked by a sturdy-looking, ageing woman with short grey hair, to make her look like Princess Diana. She replies, 'The impossible we can do today, miracles take a little longer.'

You therefore need to take on board what your hairdresser says. He or she will also think about face and body shape. I will have appraised a new client even before she gets in the chair to work out her face and body shape. Thinking about your body is important because certain hair lengths can make you look heavier or taller than you are. If you are thinking of going shorter, before you go for the snip, stand in front of a mirror and get a friend to hold your hair at different heights, so both of you can see the overall effect.

Style leaders: Jennifer Aniston, Jennifer Lopez

Thinking about your body is important because certain hair lengths can make you look heavier or taller than you are.

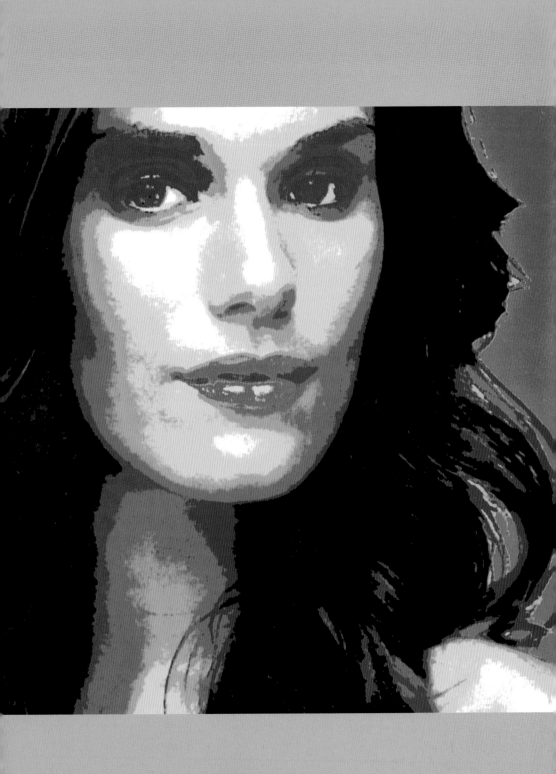

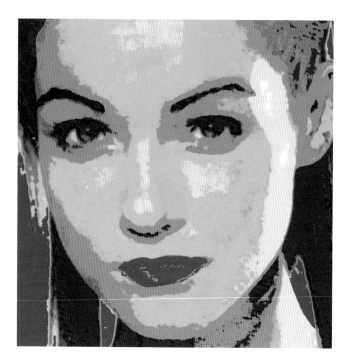

Heart

You can have your pick of literally any style – long or short, layered or blunt, straight or curly. Change your style with any fashion whim you want.

Face shape

Face shape is also an essential consideration in any restyling and something your hairdresser will have been trained to consider. We normally talk about heart, round, square, oval and long, and there are certain styles and lengths that suit particular face shapes.

Round

A layered cut or soft, feathered style will tend to suit you. Try to avoid any width in the hair around the sides of your face – this will accentuate the roundness.

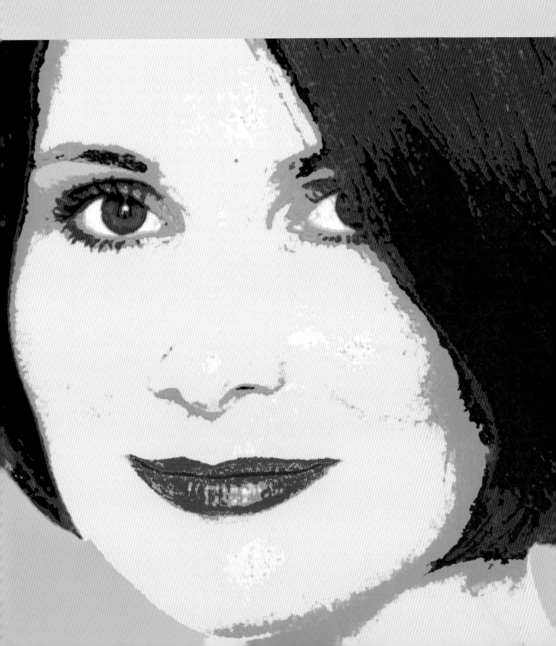

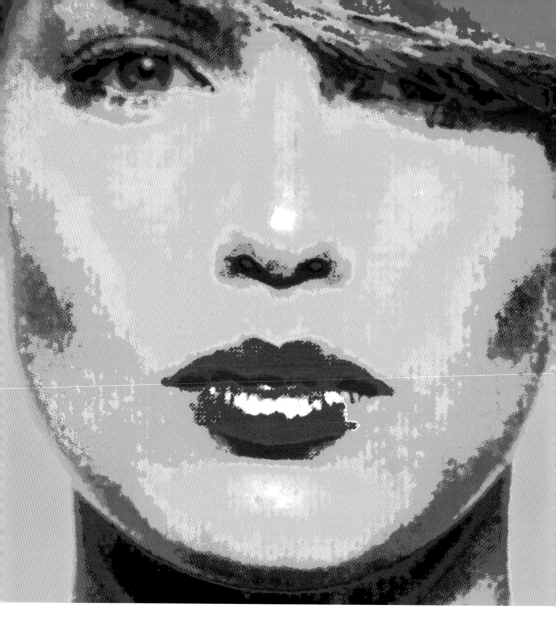

Square

Longer length, grown-out gamine crops look great on square faces, as do layered bobs with wisps around the face to soften the angles. Long layers add body which flatters your face. Avoid really close crops or severe, slicked-back styles.

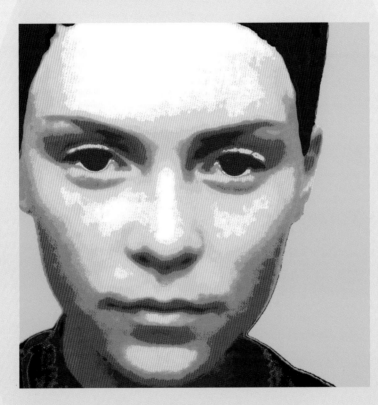

Oval

You can carry off most styles. Wild curls and big, tousled hair will set your face shape off well, as will layered styles that add volume.

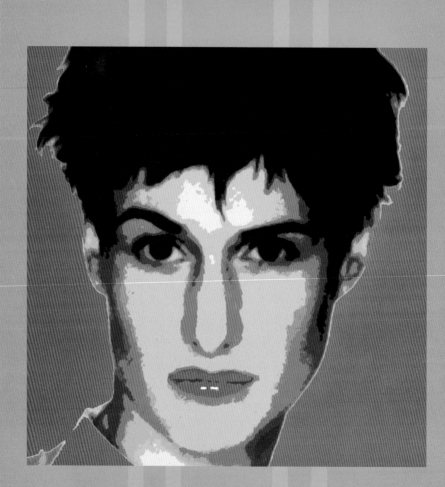

Long

Short hair can be a disaster but strangely, medium or long hair pinned up looks great. A good rule of thumb is not to cut the hair level to above the bottom of the chin.

Cutting techniques

When you see your hairdresser cutting your hair without straight lines or using a razor don't panic! Since the '60s when the clean lines of the geometric cut were introduced, hairdressers have been constantly reinventing new techniques to create movement and help the hair fall in all manner of different styles and in harmony with your natural hair. The use of the razor, which was shunned for many years, was reinvented in the late '90s. Previously used for thinning, it's now used for feathering and creating movement on the straightest of hair, cutting from the ends. My creative team coined the phrase 'Razor Behaviour' which has been adopted by stylists around the world. Your stylist may choose to cut your hair wet or dry, according to your hair type and the style you're going for. If you fancy cutting hair at home though, it's best to stick just to trimming your fringe.

Useful terms

Slide cutting	Layering in a freehand way, seemingly at random
Texturizing	Chopping into the ends of the hair
One length	All hair is cut to a single outline shape
Layering	Hair is cut at 45% to various lengths
Graduation	Gradual build up of thickness or weight in an area of the hair (classic example: the Wedge)

Partings

Increasingly, partings are used as a fashion accessory to your hairstyle. You can radically change your appearance by changing the position, depth or angle of your parting. Your hairdresser may instinctively change your parting to enhance a facial quality. Don't be afraid to ask for a hairstyle that allows you to alter your parting. It can be good for your hair to move it occasionally.

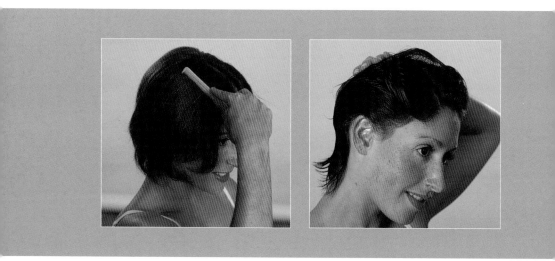

love your hair

To find your parting, comb your hair directly backwards away from your forehead. Then place the palm of your hand on the crown of your head and gently push it forward. The hair will rise up and then fall in its natural parting position.

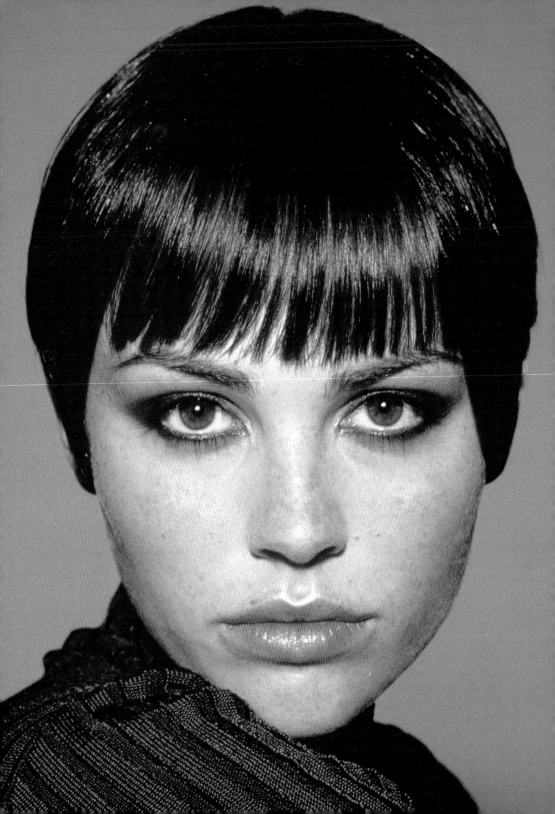

If you do have a fringe, keep it at the optimum height with regular trims. Hold the scissors vertically and snip into the hair. Avoid taking out big chunks by keeping the action small and precise.

Fringes/bangs

I love fringes. They can change the way you look, giving your face a different dimension.

If you have a high forehead or a widow's peak (cowslick), fringes are a must. But they don't have to be blunt and sit on the eyebrow. Short, chubby fringes are funky, while jagged lines are easy to trim and excellent for drawing attention to the eyes.

If you have a straight fringe divide it into thin sections and hold them back with a clip. Dampen it slightly, place a piece of tissue behind the hair so you don't cut off your eyebrows, and slowly snip across the line. Continue with each section until you have finished.

If you want to try a fringe for the first time, I would recommend you visit your hairdresser. If you've got long hair, you can see if you'd look good by putting your hair in a ponytail and holding the ends over your forehead to mimic one.

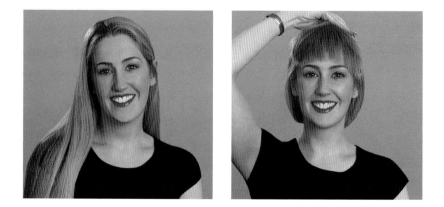

if you've never had a fringe it can be hard to imagine what you would look like with your face framed

Extensions

These are a brilliant way to change your image instantly or grow your hair out. They are available in monofibre or real hair. Both need replacing every 12 weeks. They are washable, but do take some getting used to. Many salons now offer the service. A must for international celebrities at the Oscars and MTV Awards!

PROS	CONS
Adds volume	Knots or joins can be
Adds length	uncomfortable
Helps you grow your hair during	If put in incorrectly, can fracture
that inbetween stage	root of hair permanently
Is not permanent	
Is not damaging (when done correctly)	

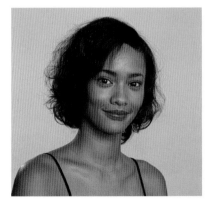 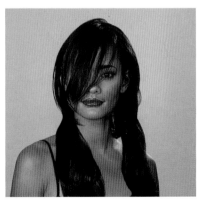

the hair is mid-length before extensions are professionally added

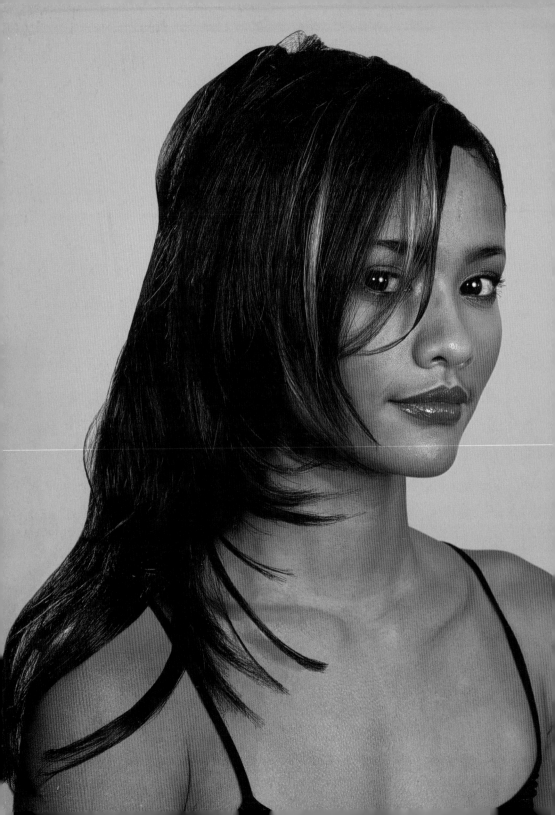

Got to be somewhere at a moment's notice and there's no time to get in a restyle at the salon?

same hair, new look'

There are many things you can do to brighten up your hair and make yourself feel glamorous.

Simple tricks

Begin with a conditioning treatment to make it more manageable and look better.

Go for the sleek and smooth look with a careful blow-dry and some serum.

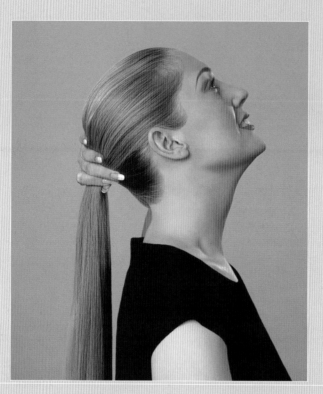

Perfect ponytail

If you're tying your hair up in a ponytail, tilt your head backwards. This way you'll gather all the hair at once and it won't bunch at the back of the neck.

angle your head backwards for the perfect ponytail

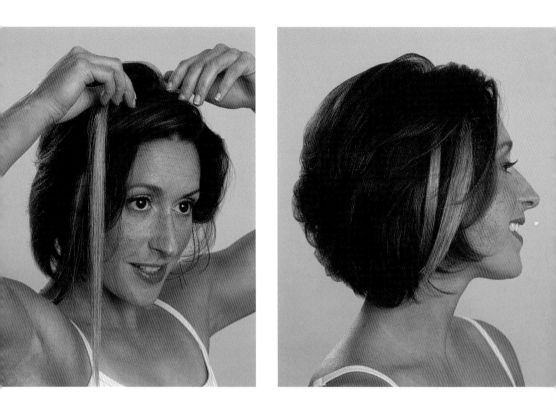

A splash of colour

Brighten up the colour with a wash-in, wash-out colour. Don't rush a permanent
or temporary colour, if it goes wrong, you'll have to stay home.

Sneak off to the High Street to pick up some temporary colour extensions to
add a bit of vibrant colour when you flick your head.

clip in the extensions close to the scalp, hiding
the clips under your own hair

trim the extensions to your own hair line for a
simple but effective new look

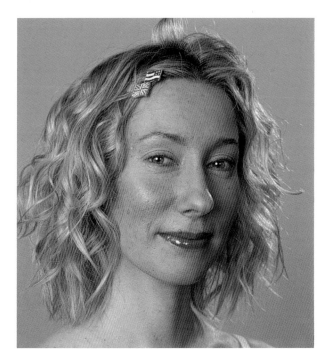

Accessorize

All that glistens could be in your hair. Try some crystal clips to add sparkle, or even some glitter spray.

False ponytails and hairslides are often used on the catwalks and are great for quick changes or detailing an outfit.

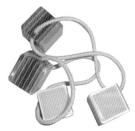

clips and hair accessories are a
simple way to adapt your look

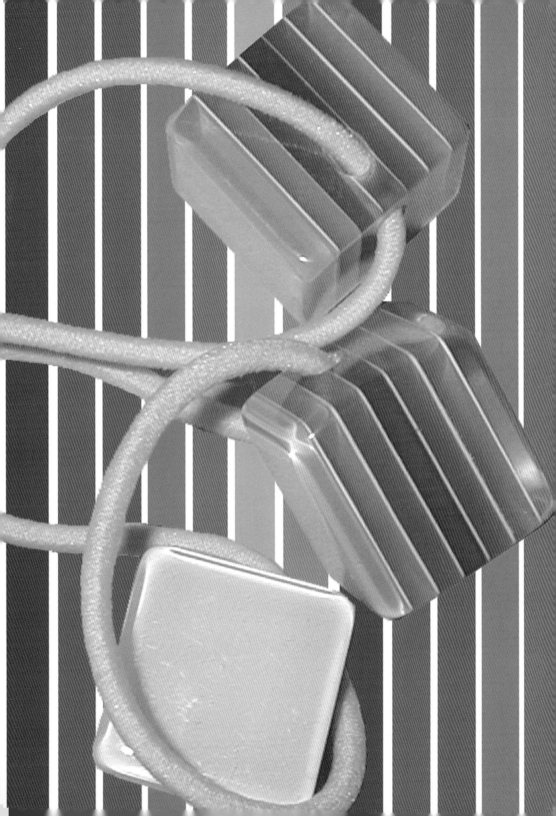

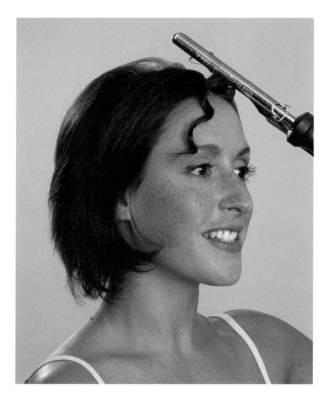

Get shape-shifting

A good tip to energize straight or wavy hair is to add three or four ringlet curls using hot tongs. Shake your hair free with your fingers and then randomly tong sections of hair. To finish, run one or two drops of serum through your hair for a stunning tousled look.

one ringlet at a time, curls tonged into moussed hair will last the night!

love your hair

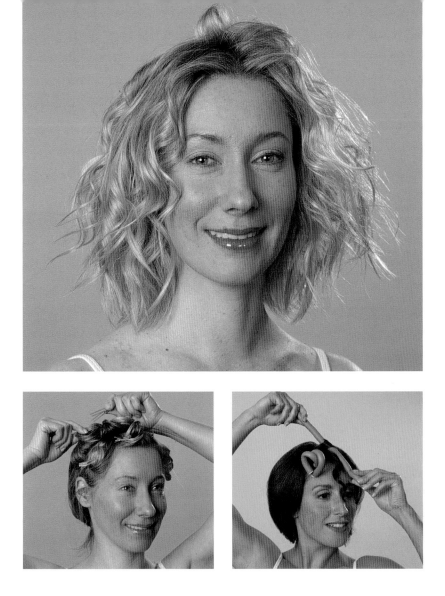

Overnight curls

Bendy rollers are an easy way to curl your hair. Put into damp hair that has mousse or a similar product in it. Dry with a diffuser or leave in overnight.

you can sleep in scrunchees for wild party curls the next morning

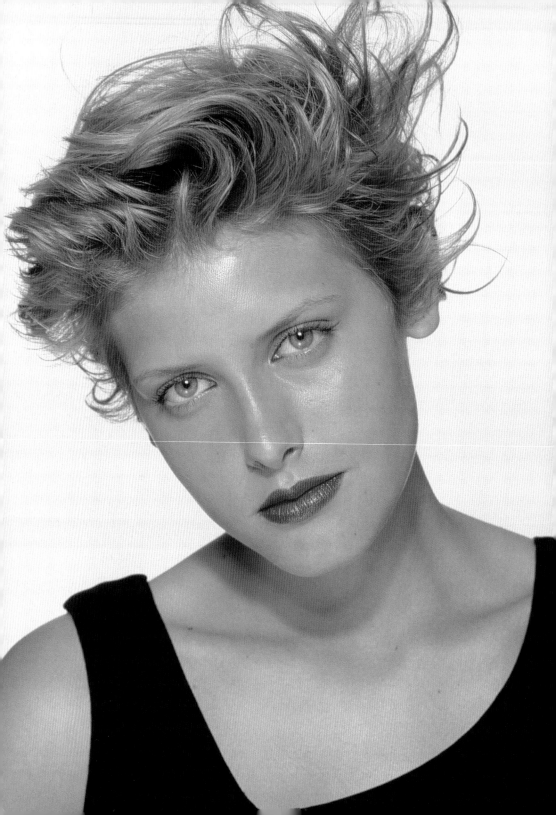

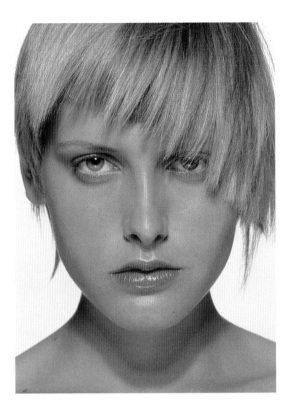

Give your hair a lift with a quiff

The hairstyle on the left is the same haircut as the one shown above, yet the finished result is radically different. To give this type of change to your style apply the mousse at the root and midlength of your hair. Blow-dry, using your fingers to lift and pull against the natural direction of the hair. Also gently scrunch the bulk of your hair when drying. Repeat the process once or twice until your hair has permanent volume. To finish, use a smoothing cream or shine product sparingly to give definition and shine.

create movement in the hair by gelling up before blow-drying

Cultivate your curls

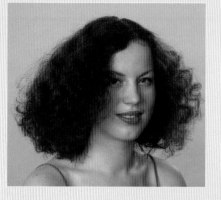

It's natural for curly or wavy hair to frizz but most of us are looking for ways to escape it.

Perfect, lasting curls like these can be achieved with the right finishing products and the special care that curly hair needs.

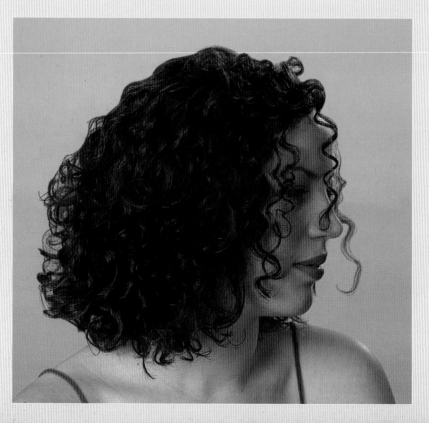

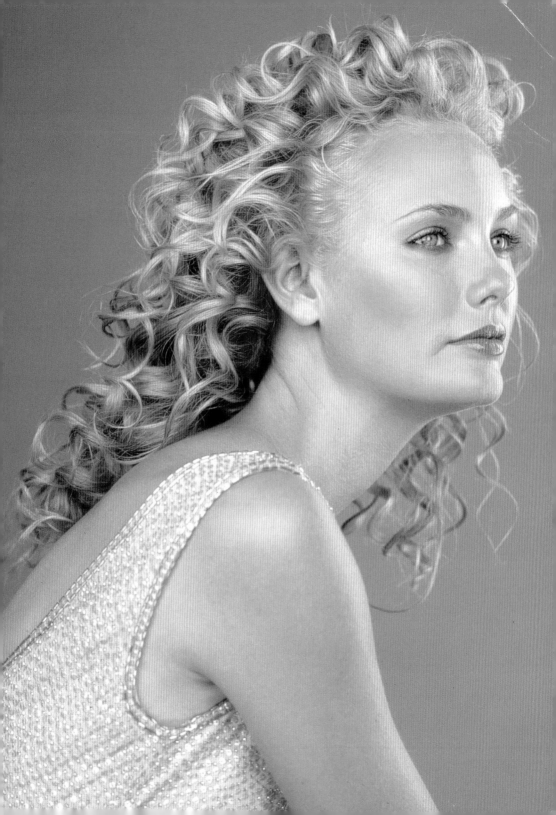

Step-by-step chignon

1   Tie your hair back in a ponytail.

2   Pull the ponytail through its own roots and pull down to create a 'twist' of hair either side of the hair band.

3   Thread the free end of hair back through the space between the two 'twists'.

4   Pull through and finally tuck the free ends under and pin to secure.

If you've no time to wash your hair, put it up. But don't go for a complicated look that you've never tried before. It's better to go for a loose chignon than waste time experimenting.

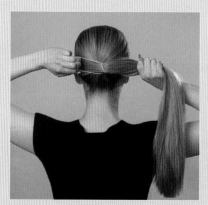 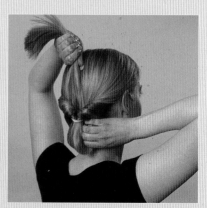

   love your hair

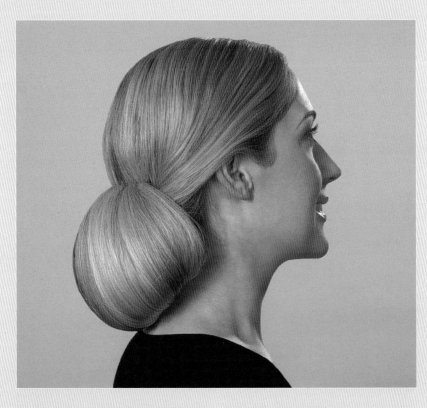

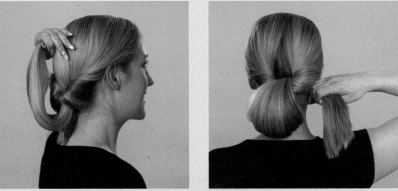

same hair, new look   87

Go straight!

1 Concentrate on perfecting the blow-dry, one section at a time.

2 After blow-drying, use straightening irons to achieve kink-free perfection.

3 The transformation from corkscrew curls to sleek and straight creates a sophisticated look with dramatic impact.

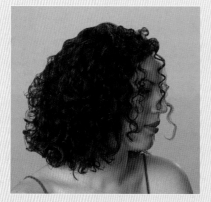 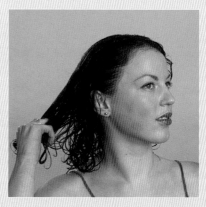

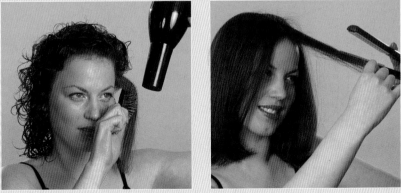

same hair, new look

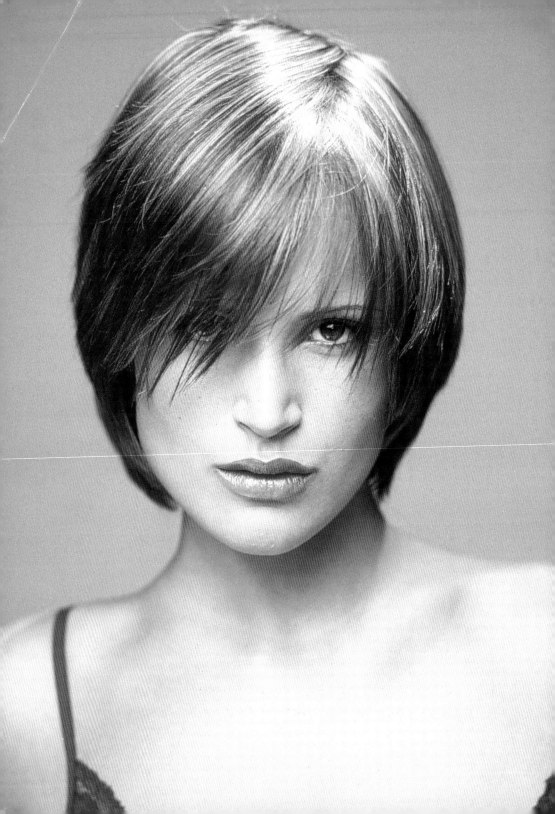

Using chemicals to change hair, such as in colour, straightening or perming can be a minefield.

get
technical

Let me tell you an old hairdresser's joke. Do you know why home colouring is called home colouring?

Because you have to stay home after doing it!

Using chemicals to change hair, such as in colour, straightening or perming, can be a minefield. There is so much choice and so much potential for things to go horribly wrong. However don't panic, I'm going to be your navigator. By the time you finish this chapter, you'll be able to have a lot of fun with colour and get some great effects yourself. You'll also know when to hotfoot it down to your favourite salon to have it done professionally. As a rule, I don't advise doing any permanent colour or perming work to hair at home because of the disasters we so often have to put right at the salon. However, it's a fact of life that many people choose to colour and perm their own hair. There are loads of fabulous, easy-to-use semi-permanent colours available and I'm also going to show you how you can straighten your hair with the minimum of damage, but I'll be upfront with you about perming for curls. It's difficult and often goes wrong. If you **must** do it yourself, have a friend assist you.

Colour

Attitudes to colour have changed dramatically over the past decade or so. We should make the most of it. Adding a few highlights, going a bit blonder or tinting it red is an excellent way to rev up your look. It makes you go 'wow', rather than just 'okay' because it's as important as make-up in making you feel gorgeous and sexy. And most of my clients agree.

Some are doing it to cover grey, others to add depth, and even more just to add a bit of interest. However you use it, it will make you feel great.

The big c

There aren't any definitive studies that have linked permanent hair colouring to cancer, but there is an element of concern which you need to think about. The excellent formulations and high-quality products used by the manufacturers, plus the awareness about cancer-inducing ingredients has lessened the risk in my view. But I reckon avoiding long-term use of all-over tints where the product is on the scalp is a wise move just in case there is a latent risk, and try to avoid permanent colour that touches the scalp during pregnancy.

love your hair

Adding a few highlights, going a bit blonder or tinting it red is an excellent way to rev up your look.

But where do you start? It can be a bit scary choosing colour for the first time. The most common one is trying to go light from dark, panicking and then trying to go back to dark. Probably every other month my stylists will see a client who has done just that. The first time she washed her hair after doing the colour, the dark tint washed right out leaving her with green hair. She then has to go to the salon to have it corrected.

Top tips for going for colour

- Ask your hairdresser for his or her opinion, especially if your hair is long. You need the advice of professionals if you want a drastic colour change, and consultations with a technician are free, even if you decide to do it yourself at home.
- Lots of salons will sell you a colour wash that matches your new colour and which can be used between appointments to brighten your hair. This is better than trying to choose one off a supermarket shelf, where the quality is great, but the colours limited.
- Home-use semi-permanent colours are risk free as they wash out.
- Think about skin tone. If you are after a natural look, you don't want your hair to clash with your skin.
- Collect pictures of colours you like and compare them to the pictures on the products or the colours on your hairdresser's colour chart.
- Consider your wardrobe and make-up, you may need to invest in some new clothes and lipstick.
- Always do a strand test beforehand to check the colour and your sensitivity to the product. You could be one of the 1-in-100 that is allergic to para-dyes, an ingredient used in many hair colours.

If you want a drastic colour change go to a professional.

- A few highlights or lowlights at your salon are inexpensive and a perfect introduction to hair colour.
- Having a small amount of streaks or a temporary colour will help build your confidence before completely taking the plunge.

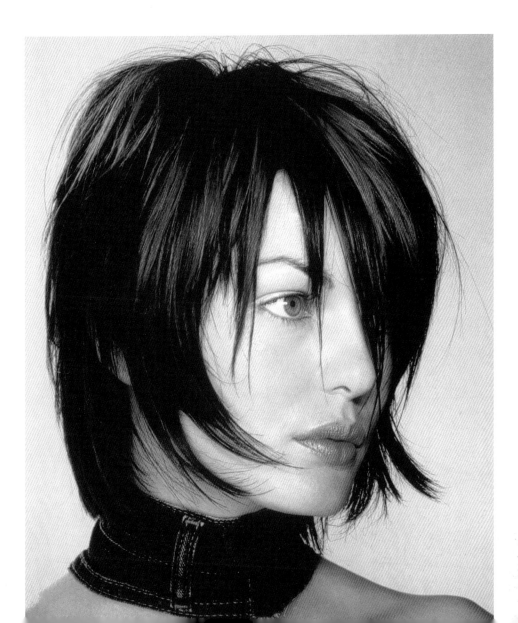

Permanent

This is by far the most popular treatment simply because it lasts longer and covers grey, but you do have to get your roots touched up regularly (every 4 to 6 weeks).

Permanent tints work by putting pigments into the hair shaft – melanin for the darker shades of brown and black and pheomelanin for red and yellow shades. But be careful, many are made from para-dyes which some people are allergic to, leading to irritation and burning. So do a skin test first. If it itches, seek out a product that doesn't contain para-dyes. Most good hairdressers will insist on this.

Tints contain a small amount of peroxide and ammonia, which get the pigment into the hair. These can be harsh on the hair. For this reason, you must touch up roots rather than go for all-over tints every time. The dyes have tiny molecules which penetrate the cuticle and enter the cortex with the help of the ammonia. Once inside, the hydrogen peroxide releases oxygen which makes the small molecules join together to create larger molecules that are too big to escape from the cortex. The result is colour that will last until you cut it off.

PROS	CONS
Permanent colour	Can damage the hair
Covers grey	Roots need retouching every 4 to 6 weeks
Lots of colours to choose from	Colour, especially reds, can fade
	May cause allergic reaction

Lightening Hair Colour

This is another permanent treatment which uses hydrogen peroxide to decolour the hair. It penetrates into the hair shaft, by means of the ammonia which lifts the cuticles, and once inside effectively zaps the pigment, making it lighter. It can go as light as you want. Again this can be a harsh treatment, so gentle aftercare is essential. You can go up to two shades lighter without bleaching.

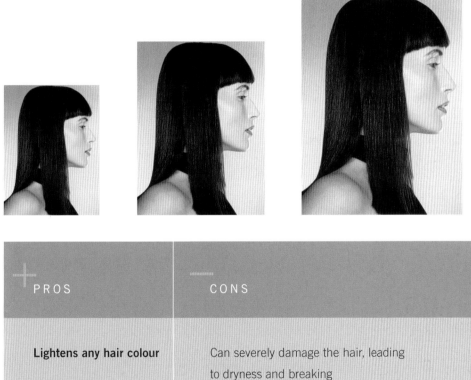

PROS	CONS
Lightens any hair colour	Can severely damage the hair, leading to dryness and breaking
Can be used in colour correction	Will need to be retouched for root growth every 4 to 6 weeks
	Can irritate the skin

Do not bleach if:

Your hair is already colour-treated, over-processed or damaged

You have cuts on your scalp (it is very painful)

Your hair is coated with a metallic substance such as hair-colour restorers

Semi-permanent

This method uses a much milder approach because it has no peroxide or ammonia to help the dye penetrate the cortex. Instead, it is absorbed into the cuticle layer and into the cortex where it sits until it is gradually washed away after a number of washes. Depending on the strength of the product, it will last 6 to 8 weeks or 10 to 20 washes, fading with each wash. The ones that last longer may have para-dyes so read the label carefully if you are doing it at home.

PROS	CONS
Good range of colours available	Washes out quickly
Won't damage the hair	Can't lighten hair
No commitment	Can lead to build up on the hair
Adds shine and gloss	
Little or no regrowth	

Demi-permanent

There is also a deposit-only treatment which does have a small amount of peroxide, but no ammonia. This is demi-permanent, half way between permanent and semi-permanent. It won't lighten or change the pigment, but it will deposit colour into the hair shaft, enhancing your natural colour and covering grey. You probably won't have regrowth because you have only added more pigment rather than changed it, and it is kinder on your hair than permanent varieties. But it won't last much longer than a semi-permanent (approximately 20 washes).

+ PROS	— CONS
Enhances colour 80%	Washes out
Covers grey	Won't lighten hair
Minimum root regrowth	

Temporary

This technique simply coats the hair with colour, which will wash out after a few shampoos. It is brilliant if you want to test a colour before taking the plunge with some more permanent effects or to liven up your hair for a special night out. And it does this without harming the hair.

PROS	CONS
Doesn't damage hair	Won't cover grey
No commitment	Washes out quickly (6 to 8 washes)
No regrowth	Won't lighten hair
Makes hair very shiny	

Natural hair colour

Over the past decade we have become much more concerned with our health and the environment. The cosmetics industry has recognized this. It has started to look for natural alternatives to chemicals. Henna has been a long-standing staple for hair colouring, but there are other alternatives now, although none are completely natural so read the labels carefully. Most will have some chemical ingredient, otherwise the colour would simply run down your face in the rain, just like your mascara. Also, because it doesn't penetrate the cortex, natural colour will not cover grey completely or allow you to change the shade of your hair drastically. If you want to go blonder or even much darker, you will need to use a chemically-enhanced product.

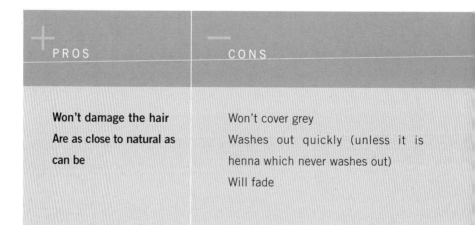

PROS	CONS
Won't damage the hair **Are as close to natural as** **can be**	Won't cover grey Washes out quickly (unless it is henna which never washes out) Will fade

Henna is still the only 100% natural way to colour hair. It comes from the leaves of the *Lawsonia inermis* plant, and colours by thickly coating the hair shaft. It will be with you for a long time and you won't be able to add any other pigments until it has grown out.

The techniques used to apply colour will also affect the overall finish of the hair. Single-application tints will give the hair colour, but not necessarily depth. If you want a more texturized look then you need highlights and lowlights which are done using foils or, in some salons, a cap.

Highlights and lowlights

Highlights are lighter than your natural colour, while lowlights are darker. This is probably the singularly most popular form of hair colouring and the effect is amazing. But it needs to be done by a skilled professional, not the junior in the salon or worse, your Mum at home. **If you are thinking of having highlights, visit your salon.**

Fashion colouring

For this to work, you need a highly talented and skilled technician who is confident as well as creative. Each salon will have their own names for these techniques. The looks will change seasonally.

Home alone

The majority of us are still colouring at home because of cost and convenience. But you must be careful. Home tints can be stronger than salon ones and are mixed for a wide range of colours. This means they may be harsher on your hair than in-salon varieties and the colour on the box may not match the end result you are left with. Your choice of colours is also limited.

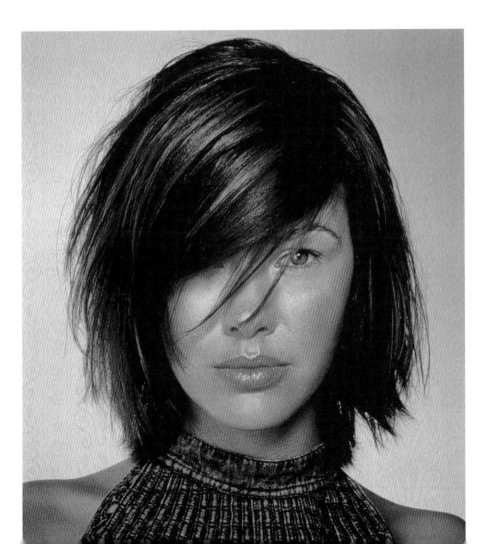

if you do home-colour follow this advice:

- Only use semi-permanent treatment at first. If you use permanent and it goes wrong, you could find your inexpensive box of dye costing you ten times the amount at the salon in colour correction. With semis, if you do get it wrong you can wash it out again.

- Choose the colour carefully. Opt for a lighter shade than the manufacturers say because it's always darker than they indicate. Check it against your skin tone to see if it suits you.

- Read the instructions twice and then follow them to the letter.

- Don't skip the strand test because you want it done for that night. What if it goes wrong? You'll be sitting in with a hat on instead of dining out. Also you may have an allergy and you could end up with an irritated scalp or worse.

- Never mix products in case you end up with a harmful chemical reaction.

- Make sure your watch is working before you start. Timing is everything with these products.

- Have someone help you to avoid patches at the back of your head.

- Rub Vaseline around the hair line to limit staining on your skin.

- Put it on reasonably clean, dry hair, but not freshly washed hair. The sebum will help protect the scalp from the dye.

- Time it exactly and then wash thoroughly with a gentle shampoo and then condition. (Always follow the manufacturer's instructions.)

Choosing a colour

Now that you know all about how the tints and lighteners work and what effects are achieved by what techniques, you have to think about what colour to go for. You should give this careful consideration, bearing in mind that skin tone is also a factor as certain colours tend to suit certain tones.

Colour indications to complement your skin tone

SKIN TONES	SUGGESTIONS
Cool – pale, ivory	Soft warm colours, pink, beiges
Warm	Terracotta, autumn shade, blueberry, red
Olive	Cooler colours, pale brunettes, chocolate, damson
Neutral	Can have most colours, dependent on personal style and season

Reds

The biggest and only problem with reds up until now is that the colour faded quicker than other tints because of the size of the molecules. However with the technological advances in colour that are happening all the time, the new reds are much less volatile. They won't fade as quickly and the range of shades is inspiring.

Blondes

It seems everyone, and not just the gentlemen, prefer blondes. But while blondes may have more fun, there is a downside. They are often considered dizzy and silly. Jerry Hall summed up the attitude to blondes perfectly when she said, 'Underneath this dizzy blonde, there's one very smart brunette.' Yet more women go blonde than any other shade. If you opt for sunny streaks or a platinum bob, you have to be careful of a few things. Smoking can turn your hair a nasty shade of yellow, while swimming in chlorinated water can turn your hair green. Lightening is also one of the most damaging treatments, so be careful with washing and over-doing the process.

Brunettes

This is the most versatile of all colours in the hair palette. It can be darkened, lightened and shaded quite easily and with the minimum of damage. Women with this colour are often considered more sensible and natural, while it's much easier to get a glossy finish on lovely dark hair. When I think of brunettes, Catherine Zeta Jones and Cindy Crawford spring to mind, with their thick luscious locks.

Grey

You will need to opt for a permanent solution. You also have to consider skin tone carefully as you go grey. A brown colour may not work for covering grey, even if you were originally a brunette. It could be too dark or too harsh against your skin. Many women find that lighter colours are very flattering.

Remember breaking the rules can have a stunning effect, but do seek the advice of a professional colourist first.

Caring for coloured hair

Once your hair is coloured, you have to treat it differently. It needs care and attention to make sure it stays in tip-top condition. This means washing it with a gentle shampoo, preferably aimed at chemically-treated hair, followed by a conditioner. Use an intensive conditioner every few weeks to help boost the shine and ensure it doesn't get too dry. Your colour could fade so reduce the frequency of washes to twice a week and wear a swimming cap when you go swimming, as chlorine can turn your lovely highlights an unpleasant green.

Colour correction

Colour correction is a job of a professional. The table to your right should give some indication of why your colour has not worked and hints on what steps to take next. Don't panic!

Incorrect colour

DISASTER	CAUSE	TIP
Ends are darker than roots	Older hair is more porous	Try again, but this time ends need to be conditioned beforehand, or put colour on for shorter time or use lighter shade on the length
Hair is darker than planned	Sometimes manufacturers products come out darker than indicated, hair is more porous	Try repeat washing
Colour is uneven	Could be hair is damaged and more porous, or it may be badly applied	Reapply to patchy areas first, before doing the rest of the hair
It hasn't covered your grey	Used the wrong product	Check label to see how much grey it will cover. You may have to opt for a permanent tint
Colour is fading too quickly	Hair is too porous, damaged or grey	Try boosting it with a temporary or semi-permanent
You hate the colour	Bad choice	Call your hairdresser
Hair meltdown	The hair loses all elasticity because it has been over-processed and can feel like sludge when wet	Avoid moisturizing products, look for ones that strengthen and rebuild the hair instead. Seek professional help

Confidence to curl

Do you gaze longingly at women with voluminous curly hair or are you one of those people who wakes every morning to a halo of ringlets and wish desperately you had a straight, sleek style? It is possible to set and dress your hair so that you can have these looks, but it can take ages, so many simply opt for the perm or relaxant. Both work in similar ways.

Perming

One of the main problems with perms over the past few years is the word. It immediately conjures up images of frizzy, dried-up hair which breaks easily and contrasts horribly with the straight virgin hair growing at the root. Recent research has found that perming is directly connected to three client phobias – it's unfashionable, it damages the condition and it means commitment. But perms aren't as out-of-date as they have been, nor do they damage hair as much and, believe it or not, some aren't even permanent anymore.

However, in response to the negative image perms have, the manufacturers have started using different vocabulary. You'll hear the terms form, texturizing, creative movement and wave.

Perms still work by chemically-altering the internal structure of the hair. First, a wave lotion is applied and then rinsed off. This is followed by a neutralizing lotion that stops the chemical reaction and sets the new structure in place permanently. It's the same process that's been used since the 1940s and the introduction of the cold wave.

However, radical advances have been made with traditional perming products so that the risk of damage is limited. Each manufacturer has developed a series of products for a variety of situations. Wella has developed an intelligent perm that scans the hair to detect variations in the hair structure, enabling it to direct the active perming lotion and conditioning ingredients to where the hair needs it most. While L'Oréal's Dulcia range only works for a precise time, ensuring the hair can't be over-processed.

The manufacturers are also developing products to help amend perms. Schwarzkopf has the Natural Styling Curl Softener which can be used to soften curls if a perm is too tight.

The new wave

The most radical development over the past few years has been the introduction of semi-permanent perms, such as L'Oréal's Animatic, Aveda's demi perms and Wella's Perform Hairscan L, all in-salon treatments. These products bring volume to the hair without many of the risks associated with traditional perming. And they can give curl or texture. However, they don't last very long, they tend to create waves rather than curls and they don't work well on hair longer than below the nape. But otherwise, they are fun.

Home perming

- Always read the instructions through at least twice.
- Put a watch close by and make sure you don't leave the lotions on a minute longer than the instructions say.
- Get everything ready beforehand.
- Work out a pattern for the curlers and wind them very carefully. Too tight and you could lose your hair, too loose and the whole process will be pointless.
- Undo a curler and test the curl for buoyancy.
- Don't shampoo the hair for two to three days as the process continues even after you have washed off the products.

Permed hair requires the same careful approach as coloured hair: gentle shampoos, specially formulated for colour-treated hair, and lots of conditioning treatments.

Do not perm/relax hair if:

It has been colour-treated

It is weak and damaged

It is susceptible to breakage

Incorrect Perm Result

DISASTER	CAUSE	TIP
Curl uneven	Lotion misapplied and hasn't been able to penetrate from the root to the tip	Get advice from your hairdresser to see if hair is strong enough to be re-permed and then let him or her do it. **Don't do it at home**
Curls too tight and frizzy	Product left on too long or incorrect winding of rollers	Relax by blow-drying and heavy conditioning or call the salon to see if they have a curl relaxer
Hair falling out in clumps	Roller wound too tight, hair combed badly during relaxant phase	Go to your hairdresser immediately, the only solution may be short hair
Hair meltdown	The hair looses all elasticity because it has been over-processed and can feel like sludge when wet. Avoid moisturizing products, look for ones that strengthen and rebuild the hair instead	Avoid moisturizing products, look for ones that strengthen. Seek professional help

Chemical straightening

The products available nowadays, especially those for Afro hair, are excellent and have been well designed for home use. Although it uses the same process as perming, because there are no rollers and twisting involved, you can do a great job at home. But you still have to be sensible.

Always read the instructions twice.

Follow them to the letter.
Keep a close eye on time.
Avoid using clips.
Don't wash your hair for two days because the process continues even after the chemicals have been removed.
Don't use metal combs.

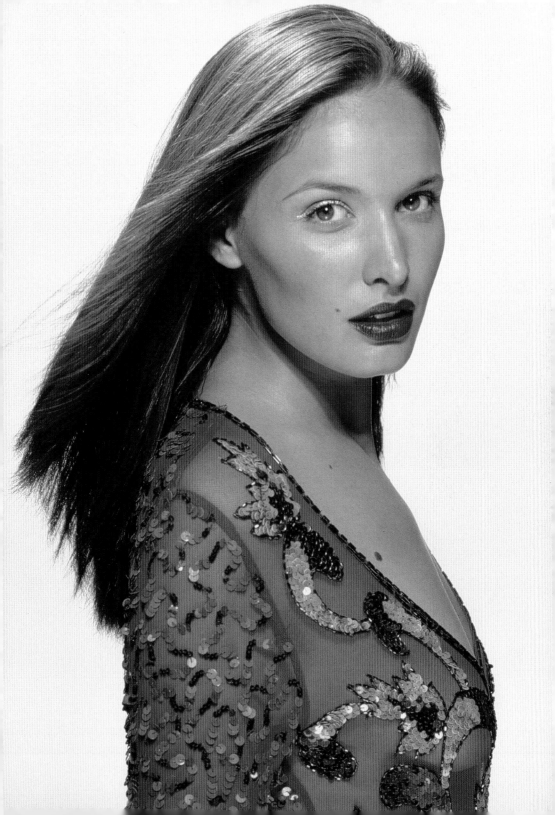

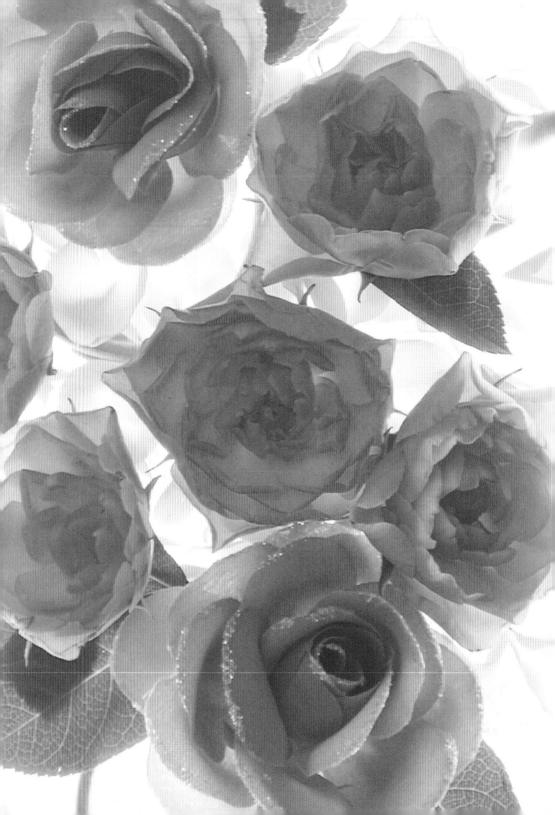

Hair is a wonderful material. It is strong and resilient, especially if you don't abuse it.

hair
concerns

Hair protects your scalp, enhances your looks and makes you feel good. However, there are some common disorders like dandruff and head lice that need special treatment. Others are more serious and it's advisable to see your doctor or a trichologist.

Hair loss

Probably the most upsetting scalp condition a woman can suffer from is hair loss. Known by the collective name of alopecia, this is no longer a male-only problem. Stress, pollution, eating habits, ill health and medication are all contributing to the new phenomenon of female baldness. It happens when the follicle is damaged and stops producing keratin. The existing hair will fall out, but no new hair will grow. It is devastating.

According to Elizabeth Steel, who founded Hairline International, the Alopecia Patients' Society, after losing her hair, up to a third of the whole population suffers hair loss, and thousands of them are women.

The most important thing you can do if you notice you are losing more hair than normal (typically a person loses 100 hairs a day) is to consult a doctor. The follicles may have only stopped working temporarily and treatment may get them active again. Improving your diet, taking a mineral supplement, reducing stress and taking a hormone treatment could all help. There are also drug remedies such as Regaine, which contains minoxidil (a drug used for high blood pressure). One of its side effects is increased hair growth. However, when you stop using it, the positive effects will also stop.

Trichologists are experts on scalp health. They have treatments not available from your doctor or hairdresser.

love your hair

Variants of alopecia

ANDROGENIC ALOPECIA

This is the medical name for pattern baldness commonly associated with men. Increasing numbers of women are developing it as well. Stress is considered a major contributor. Hormone treatment can slow down and even stop this sort of hair loss.

ALOPECIA AREATA

This is where patches of hair fall out for no apparent reason. They are often associated with auto-immune disorders. Steroid creams can help, or more extreme treatments include PUVA used to treat psoriasis, a light/drug combination therapy where UVA rays are used with a light-sensitive drug.

ALOPECIA TOTALIS

This is a term used when all the hair on the head is lost, including eyebrows and eyelashes.

TRACTION ALOPECIA

Pulling back the hair too tightly, too often can lead to this sort of hair loss, so watch out if you put your hair in tight braids or ponytails.

POSTPARTUM ALOPECIA

Having a baby and breast-feeding sends your hormones into overload and this can affect hair. During pregnancy, your hair will be retained but can then fall out after the birth. It usually grows back within a few months.

TRICHOTILLOMANIA

This is a condition where people are compelled to pull out the hair on their scalp, eyebrows and even eyelashes. Sufferers normally have some sort of emotional problem and can be helped through counselling, anti-depressant drugs and hypnosis.

Dandruff

For some people the option of wearing classic black is just not on. No one wants to advertise their dandruff by wearing a colour that will immediately show up those tiny white flakes as they flutter down. While not all flaky scalps are caused by dandruff, it is a common problem. According to Gallup, 30% of all 25 to 39 year olds are affected by the condition.

It is thought to be caused by a microscopic fungal yeast called *pityrosporum ovale* which is present in small amounts on everyone's scalp, but is more prevalent on the scalp of a dandruff sufferer. It is caused when the scalp becomes irritated and the skin cells start to overproduce. The yeast then grows more rapidly and the cells clump together producing the familiar flakes of dandruff. It can be exacerbated by environment or hormone levels, however, it is not infectious and is not the result of bad hygiene or stress. Tell-tale signs are small white loose flakes on the scalp, a dry scalp and an itchy scalp.

If you suddenly find you have these symptoms, don't dash out to buy the treatment shampoos. Try a moisturizing shampoo, conditioner or scalp treatment in case it is simply dry skin. If it persists, then try the anti-dandruff products.

SEBORRHOEIC DERMATITIS

This is a more extreme version, where the fungal yeast is in even higher quantities. This is particularly common in men between the ages of 20 and 40. It can be aggravated by stress, but it can also be inherited. The tell-tale signs are large, greasy, yellowish scales which stick to the scalp and inflammation, plus a tendency to also affect the forehead, eyebrows, chest and back.

Start using an anti-dandruff shampoo. But if it is very bad, talk to your hairdresser or pharmacist to get his or her recommendation; you may need a stronger product.

Impetigo

This is caused when a bacteria enters a cut or abrasion, (usually caused through scratching). Sores will grow and develop golden scabs. Impetigo is highly infectious and will rapidly spread to other wounds. The only treatment is antibiotics, which you can take orally or as a cream.

Boils

Boils are caused by *bacteria staphylococci* entering a hair follicle or sebaceous gland. It swells up and causes a lot of pain and discomfort. Again, go to your doctor for treatment.

Lice

Lice are becoming more common as they develop immunity to the chemicals used, despite the recommendation to alternate the products available in chemists. They lay their eggs on the hair shaft which stick solid and are difficult to move. Transmission can happen between towels and hats, but the easiest way is from head-to-head contact.

There are a variety of treatments for lice. The traditional approach has been to douse the head in pesticide, with a second application seven days later. If this doesn't work, it could be because the lice are immune to that particular chemical. There are non-pesticide shampoos but these are less effective.

NIT COMBS

These are narrow-toothed combs that will catch the adult lice.

Giving your hair a comb through every three days will catch the lice as they hatch and won't give them time to breed. There are electronic combs that zap the lice as they are touched.

AROMATHERAPY OILS

These may help. Try combing a little tea tree or lavender oil diluted in a base oil through the hair. Always wash it out the next day as it makes the hair greasy.

Ringworm

Ringworm is another form of infestation, this time by a fungi that gets into the skin and causes circular patches. It doesn't just affect the scalp, but once there it can cause hair loss through itching. Treat it with an anti-fungal agent, similar to anti-dandruff lotions.

Eczema

Eczema is becoming more common, especially in children and can affect the scalp making it itchy and sore. Traditional medicines don't seem to have much effect, but Chinese herbal medicine can help, so check it out.

Psoriasis

Psoriasis is a disfiguring ailment that can affect the whole scalp or sometimes just the hairline. It happens when the outer layer of skin is missing or flakes off, leaving itchy, tender skin. Chamomile may help, but it is best to seek treatment from your GP.

Contact dermatitis

If you find your skin flares up after contact with certain products then you are probably suffering from contact dermatitis. You are probably sensitive to the shampoo and other products you are using. Try a product specially formulated for sensitive skin, which will have less additives, perfume or colouring.

Sebaceous cysts

Sebaceous cysts are unsightly little lumps that occur when keratin accumulates under the skin. They may appear on their own or in clusters, and are not normally painful or irritating, but they may get so big that you catch them with your brush or comb. It's easy to have them removed.

Health and hair

Nutrients or lack of them have a great effect on the general wellbeing of our skin and hair. It can slow down growth, cause our hair to dry out or break off or even cause it to fall out. A balanced diet really does work. Overleaf is a table of vitamins and minerals that shows what they can do for your hair health.

Feed your hair

NUTRIENT	WHAT IT DOES	SOURCES
A	Important for natural development of skin and hair; keeps the scalp healthy	Dairy products, fish oil, spinach, apricots
B	Necessary for protein metabolism and building the red blood cells that carry nutrients to different parts of the body, including the hair follicle and bulb	Meat, fish, some pulses, bananas, leafy green vegetables, dairy products and yeast extract
C	Helps absorb other nutrients necessary to body and hair; neutralizes free radicals	Citrus fruits, melon, broccoli, Brussels sprouts, tomatoes and potatoes
D	Necessary for skin and hair development	Sunshine, salmon, liver
E	Antioxidant; helps healthy tissue growth	Wheat germ, nuts, broccoli, green leafy vegetables and whole grain
Zinc	Essential for hair growth	Some nuts, wholewheat, red meat and eggs
Iron	Again essential for hair growth	Red meat, pulses, spinach

Iron and zinc are essential for healthy hair, and can even lead to hair loss if deficient, so be especially careful if you are cutting down on or cutting out meat from your diet. Compensate with lots of green leafy vegetables and pulses like lentils or beans. Another element of our diet that has been vilified in recent years is fat. We still need it in our diet because it helps us absorb the other nutrients. It's just better if it is unsaturated. **Moderation is the secret to beautiful hair.**

Water

Besides eating well, we also have to watch what we drink. About 70 per cent of the human body is made up of water and we have to keep it stocked up. So every day we should be drinking about two litres of water. It may seem a lot but it's only about eight glasses. Drinking water will hydrate the hair from the inside. Sadly, coffee, tea and alcohol don't have the same hydrating effect. In fact, they inhibit hydration so you have to keep them to a minimum.

Sleep

While what we eat influences development of our hair, what goes on around our body also affects it as well. And that means lifestyle. Lack of sleep tarnishes the healthy glow of hair as much as it affects skin, and in extreme cases can lead to hair loss.

Exercise

Exercise is good for your health, but you have to take special care of your hair, otherwise it could be damaged, particularly when swimming.

SWIMMING

When you go swimming, you saturate your hair in chlorine, which makes it dry and brittle. It can also turn coloured or highlighted hair a nasty shade of green. Wet your hair before entering the pool and put conditioner on it. It is also a good idea to wear a swimming cap.

OUTDOOR SPORTS

Outdoor sports, such as tennis or running, expose your hair to the sun's rays, potentially drying it out and making it brittle, so try wearing a baseball cap. Exercising every day can lead to frequent washing, which in turn can lead to frequent blow-drying – a major hazard. Use a protective blow-dry spray. The dry heat of a sauna can dehydrate the hair, so add conditioner to moisturize beforehand.

Tying hair back

Many clients I meet in their mid to late 20s, who have worn their hair long all their lives and now wish to change their style, have their options limited by the fineness of their front hair line and the height of their forehead. This has often been caused by what I call the 'ballet-school syndrome', where the hair has been scraped back too tightly in childhood, damaging young hair growth.

To avoid traction (pulling) alopecia, always use scrunchies rather than bands and don't pull the front hairline too tight.

Daily wear and tear

The most common form of daily wear and tear is the constant touching, fiddling, flicking and rubbing of hair, not to mention sticking pens in it. The acid on your fingers will damage the fine front hairs with constant picking and touching. And it may make your hair greasier more quickly as you move sebum along the shaft.

Age

As we age hair changes and by the time we get to our thirties and forties some hairs may begin to grow without any melanin or colour. At the same time, these grey hairs lose their elasticity and become coarser, and the sebaceous glands stop producing as much sebum. There is nothing you can do to reverse this action at the moment, although scientists are working on it, but you can cover it up with tints and highlights. The length of time a hair grows also gets shorter, so it's more difficult to grow your hair long.

Pregnancy and breastfeeding

Pregnancy and birth can also affect hair. During pregnancy some women may find their hair feels thicker. This is due to the hormones produced during pregnancy, which stop hair falling out at the normal rate. Pregnant women also have more blood coursing through their veins than normal. It circulates around the body and up to the scalp, feeding the hair. Sadly, when you have the baby, the thick, glossy hair can be lost as the scalp sheds the hair retained during the nine months. Pregnancy can also affect the type of hair you have. I have a client who has tight curly hair, but sections of her hair grew straight while she was carrying her son. After her son was born, her hair grew back curly.

Breastfeeding can also affect the condition of the hair, drying it up, as the body directs most of the nutrients towards the baby. This will return to normal once you stop feeding, but may take up to a year.

Illness

Finally, drugs and ill-health can seriously affect hair growth. Actual illness can change the hair and cause hair thinning through hormonal imbalances, while treatments such as chemotherapy, can cause rapid hair loss and baldness. In most cases the hair will grow back. There are now ice caps available for use in the chemo process, which considerably improve the chances of keeping your hair. Your doctor will be able to advise.

questions & answers

I am frequently asked
about a number of hair concerns,
so I have answered some of the more
common questions in this section.

What is dandruff? How do I tackle it?

Dandruff is a yeast. You will know if you have dandruff by the size of the flakes of dry skin – they are large. You can use an anti-dandruff shampoo to control the condition. Doctors or trichologists can prescribe an antifungal solution for persistent conditions.

I'm losing my hair; what do I do?

Hair loss is either genetic, hormonal or stress related. Many Indian women experience hair thinning; others may experience it during menopause or post-pregnancy. Visit a trichologist if this is happening. In addition to the various treatments on offer, some people suggest that a one-minute headstand (or for most of us lying on our bed and hanging your head over the end) can slow down thinning as the blood is forced into the scalp, feeding the bulb of the hair shaft.

What can I do about my split ends?

The only way to get rid of them is to cut them off. There are some products which claim to conceal them by coating the shaft and gluing the split ends together. I would advise cutting away the damage though.

Is brushing my hair good for it? I was always told you should give it 100 strokes.

Brushing the hair is good and do not be fearful of hair in the brush. You will lose between 100 and 150 hairs a day. Be careful not to tear the hair. Nothing beats a good Mason & Pearson brush. Never brush hair when it's wet, always use a comb. If you have knots and tangles, always brush from the ends upwards. You won't need 100 strokes though!

Does rubbing your hair with a silk scarf make your hair shine?

Yes it does. After brushing, gently rub it from side to side and down the length of the hair.

Does washing your hair more frequently make it greasier?

No, but frequent washing is addictive and daily washers will never settle for anything less than super-fresh hair. Conditioning is advisable for longer-length hair.

Is soft or hard water better for your hair?

Products perform differently. You may need to rethink your haircare choices when you move town. Neither damage the hair. Soft water makes the hair very soft and silky.

I've been told that I should change my brand of shampoo regularly as hair responds well to a change. Is this true?

I recommend you use a clarifying shampoo once a month. This will give you 'start-again' hair, allowing you to choose the way your hair will perform and enabling you to reassess your needs.

My hair is going grey. When should I consider colouring?

Some people like the salt-and-pepper effect as they like to feel the recognition of becoming mature and more distinguished. This is often a passing phase! You can introduce colour in such subtle ways that over a period of time your hair appears more attractive and healthy, seemingly without effort. Only a hair-dresser can achieve this subtle effect.

Is using a hot hairdryer really going to damage my hair?

Only if you hold it too close to the hair. Hold it at least 15 cm (6 inches) away.

I think I have an allergy to my shampoo. What should I do?

The word hypoallergenic is in fact pretty meaningless. Try avoiding the following ingredients, checking your hair product labels carefully, some of them are for cosmetics in general, not specifically for hair products:

2,4-Diaminophenol (and HCl)	Glyceryl Stearate
2-Bromo-2-nitropropane-1,3-diol	Isopropanolamine
BHA	m-Phenylenediamine (and Sulfate)
BHT	Methylchloroisothiazolinone
Cocamide DEA	Methylisothiazolinone
Cocamide MEA	Myristyl Alcohol
Cocamide MIPA	Oleamidopropyl Dimethylamine
Cocamidopropyl Betaine	Phenoxyethanol
DEA-Oleth-10 Phosphate	Propyl Gallate
Dihydroxyacetone (DHA)	Propylene Glycol
Glyceryl Oleate	Stearyl Alcohol

I'd really like to use a product range that hasn't been tested on animals. Have you any recommendations?

There are many product ranges in store and in salon which haven't been tested on animals. Although laws governing sale of retail products will have been adhered to for public safety, meaning that some ingredients may have been purchased by the manufacturer post testing.

I've heard that dark hair dyes can cause cancer or arthritis. Is this true?

Some research has suggested this. If you are particularly worried about the risk then avoid colouration techniques where colour comes into contact with the skin. There are safe products for sale in health stores, but they usually give limited performance. Natural henna is a notable exception.

Andrew's favourite magical haircare tools and products

Hairdressing salons, supermarkets and specialist shops have an overwhelming choice of products. Many will be good and a few will be great. What I list in the chart overleaf is by no means definitive. These are products I have tried, used and can recommend as they will do what's needed for your hair – with care.

Tools

The tools that you use on our hair can make all the difference. In general, tools that have been designed for the professional hairdresser will give the best result. As a rule of thumb choose those manufacturers that sell both to the hairdresser, and to you the consumer.

A good example is the innovative range of brushes and combs by Denman.

Andrew's favourite magical hair products

PRODUCT	CLAIM	SUITABLE FOR	SHAMPOOS
Clarifying	Start-again hair	Over-coated hair, removes product build up	KMS Clarifying, Pantene Clarifying
For curls	Encourages curl, reduces frizz	Naturally curly hair	Pantene Perfect Curls
Daily	Cleans and cares without damaging	Daily or frequent washing	Pantene Classic Care, Paul Mitchell Awapuhi
Moisturizing	Add moisture, smoothes hair shaft, feels softer	Dry, brittle hair	KMS Moisture, Schwarzkopf Bonacure, L'Oréal Kerastase
Straightening	Perfect, sleek straight hair	Catwalk perfect hair	KMS Flatout, Pantene Smooth & Sleek
Strengthening	Rebuilds hair shaft, increases elasticity	Fine, weak hair (naturally or due to chemical process)	Redken product by stylist recommendation – Protein Enriched
Swimming care	Anti-salt/chlorine	Regular swimmers	Joico Altma
Volumizing	Root life and body	For fine or limp hair, and 'big-hair' fans	Redken Fat Cat, Pantene Sheer Volume, KMS Amp-Volume

CONDITIONERS	STYLING/SPECIAL CARE	TOOLS
Joico Lite		
MOP Leave-in Conditioner	John Frieda Frizz Ease, KMS Weightless Shine, Joico Ice	Wide-toothed comb. Let it dry naturally or use a diffuser
Paul Mitchell The Conditioner, MOP Daily Conditioning, Pantene Classic Care Conditioner	Any to suit style	Dependent on style
KMS Daily Repair		
KMS Flatout, Pantene Sleek & Smooth	John Frieda Frizz Ease, Schwarzkopf Sealed Ends, MOP D. Curl	Paddlebrush by Denman, or one with big round bristles to remove wave or curl
Use a conditioner in tandem with your Redken shampoo	Pantene Strengthening Serum	Be careful with brushes and combs as they put stress on hair
Add any conditioner to damp hair before swimming	Swim hats work!	Detangle comb – wide toothed
Redken Fat Cat, Pantene Sheer Volume, KMS Amp-Volume	Text It, Osis by Schwarzkopf, Pantene Sheer Volume Root Booster, Redken Fat Cat Volume Spray	Round or bristled hair brush

Session bag
secrets

Phyto Plage by Phytologie for glamorous unkempt hair.
Silk and Groom by Kiehl's for Hollywood hair.
Talcum Power disguises excess product in an instant.

Funky
stuff

Chop 'n' change hairstyles have a huge range of products to define
and texturize. Many greats are within these ranges:

Sebastian
Osis by Schwarzkopf
Tigi
High Hair by Wella
Fudge

Household
haircare

Lavender Rinse adds shine.
Tomato Ketchup removes green in blond hair. Apply like conditioner.
Beer can be used to add volume when blow-drying.

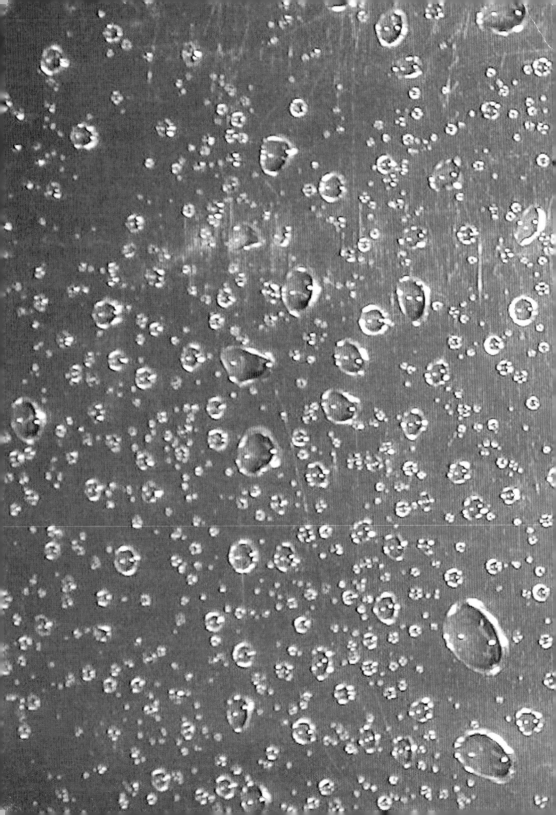

index

Andrew Jose salons are in London and Prague and new openings in capital cities are being planned. They pride themselves on the quality of their hairdressing.

The salons are centrally located and attractively designed providing an enjoyable environment with fabulous service.

Salons

London: 1 Charlotte Street W1T 1RB
tel: +44 (0)20 7323 4679

Prague: Michalska 17
Praha 1 110 00
tel: +42 02 2423 2029

Schools

The Andrew Jose Academy and Schools are located in London's Bloomsbury and Michalska Street in Prague. They teach Andrew Jose techniques and philosophy of hairdressing to hairdressers from all over the world. There are excellent courses for beginners with a high ratio of teachers to students. Nationally recognized qualifications are awarded and there is also the opportunity to become a member of the Andrew Jose association of quality hairdressers.

London: 84 Lambs Conduit Street WC1N 3LR
tel: +44 (0)20 7242 5057

Prague: Michalska 17
Praha 1 110 00
tel: +42 02 2423 2029

If you have a specific hair concern please contact us by visiting the Andrew Jose website at **www.andrewjose.com** which contains haircare information as well as:

- Salon details
- Education Information
- News

- Live Show
- Monthly prize draw to win a haircut

www.andrewjose.com

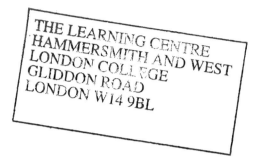